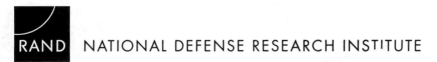
NATIONAL DEFENSE RESEARCH INSTITUTE

The Defense and Veterans Brain Injury Center Care Coordination Program

Assessment of Program Structure, Activities, and Implementation

Laurie T. Martin, Coreen Farris, Andrew M. Parker, Caroline Epley

Prepared for the Office of the Secretary of Defense

The research described in this report was prepared for the Office of the Secretary of Defense (OSD). The research was conducted within the RAND National Defense Research Institute, a federally funded research and development center sponsored by OSD, the Joint Staff, the Unified Combatant Commands, the Navy, the Marine Corps, the defense agencies, and the defense Intelligence Community under Contract W74V8H-06-C-0002.

Library of Congress Cataloging-in-Publication Data

Martin, Laurie T. (Laurie Thayer), 1974-
  The Defense and Veterans Brain Injury Center Care Coordination Program :
assessment of program structure, activities, and implementation / Laurie T. Martin,
Coreen Farris, Andrew M. Parker, Caroline Epley.
    pages cm
  Includes bibliographical references.
  ISBN 978-0-8330-8099-8 (pbk. : alk. paper)
  1. Defense and Veterans Brain Injury Center (Washington, D.C.)—Evaluation. 2.
Disabled veterans—Medical care—United States—Management. 3. Brain damage—
Patients—Rehabilitation—United States—Management. I. Farris, Coreen. II. Parker,
Andrew M. III. Epley, Caroline. IV. Title.
  RC387.5.M3697 2013
  362.4086'97—dc2   201303184

The RAND Corporation is a nonprofit institution that helps improve policy and decisionmaking through research and analysis. RAND's publications do not necessarily reflect the opinions of its research clients and sponsors.

Support RAND—make a tax-deductible charitable contribution at www.rand.org/giving/contribute.html

RAND® is a registered trademark

RAND OFFICES
SANTA MONICA, CA • WASHINGTON, DC
PITTSBURGH, PA • NEW ORLEANS, LA • JACKSON, MS • BOSTON, MA
DOHA, QA • CAMBRIDGE, UK • BRUSSELS, BE
www.rand.org

Preface

Many consider traumatic brain injury (TBI) to be the "signature wound" of operations Enduring Freedom and Iraqi Freedom. Although the majority of individuals with TBI can expect a full recovery, others require additional support services in a system that can be difficult to navigate, particularly through transitions across systems of care or permanent changes of station. In 2007, several reports emphasized the need for care coordination services specific to TBI. In response, the Defense and Veterans Brain Injury Center (DVBIC) launched the regional Care Coordination Program (CCP) to provide services to active duty service members and veterans with ongoing symptoms associated with a TBI incurred while serving in operations Enduring Freedom and Iraqi Freedom. The DVBIC viewed CCP as a natural extension of its ongoing work to support active duty service members and veterans with TBI, as well as their beneficiaries, through clinical, research, and educational programs.

Launched in 2007, CCP provides education and care coordination services to individuals with unresolved TBIs. Regional care coordinators work closely with individuals to assess their unique needs and provide recommendations for local program resources that will help to meet these needs. By design, individuals are followed for up to two years, with scheduled contacts at three, six, nine, 12, 18, and 24 months after program enrollment, to assess problem resolution and the need for additional or different services.

The purpose of this report is to assess CCP's program structure, activities, and implementation. We conducted this assessment between April and July 2012. During this assessment, we spoke with program leadership and 11 of the 14 regional care coordinators. These discussions included the following topics: program services, eligibility criteria, outreach activities, caseloads, work environments and staffing structure, barriers and facilitators of successful care coordination, perceived program benefits, and opportunities for improvement. We also analyzed the content of the DVBIC websites specific to CCP.

The contents of this report will be of particular interest to organizations related to CCP, including the Defense Centers of Excellence for Psychological Health and Traumatic Brain Injury, DVBIC, and CCP leadership. The contents of the report may also be of interest to national policymakers within the Department of Defense and the U.S. Department of Veterans Affairs. Finally, results of this assessment will be of value to other programs interested in establishing or refining similar programs across multiple systems of care.

This research was sponsored by the Defense Centers of Excellence for Psychological Health and Traumatic Brain Injury and conducted within the Forces and Resources Policy Center of the RAND National Defense Research Institute, a federally funded research and development center sponsored by the Office of the Secretary of Defense, the Joint Staff, the Unified Combatant Commands, the Navy, the Marine Corps, the defense agencies, and the defense Intelligence Community. For more information on the RAND Forces and Resources Policy Center, see http://www.rand.org/nsrd/ndri/centers/frp.html or contact the director (contact information is provided on the web page).

Contents

Figures

Tables

Summary

Between 2001 and 2011, 2.2 million service members were deployed in support of Operation Enduring Freedom (OEF) and Operation Iraqi Freedom (OIF). Improvised explosive devices have been used extensively against U.S. forces during these conflicts and have been one of the leading causes of death. Injuries among those who survive an improvised explosive device blast often include traumatic brain injuries (TBIs), which have been called the signature injury of the OEF/OIF conflict. Service members recovering from a TBI often find they must coordinate services across multiple systems of care to meet all their medical and psychological health needs. This task is difficult even for those without the cognitive challenges associated with TBI and may prove overwhelming or even impossible for those recovering from a TBI. This report focuses on a program designed to facilitate care coordination for service members and veterans recovering from a symptomatic brain injury—the Defense and Veterans Brain Injury Center (DVBIC) Care Coordination Program (CCP). CCP services bridge both the Department of Defense (DoD) and Department of Veterans Affairs (VA) systems of care, but the program is funded and overseen by DoD.

In 2007, DVBIC launched CCP to provide services to active duty, National Guard, and Reserve service members and veterans with ongoing symptoms associated with mild or moderate TBIs incurred while serving in OEF/OIF. Regional care coordinators (RCCs) are tasked with ensuring that individuals remain connected to the services they need to recover from a TBI, particularly during difficult transition points (e.g., during the transition from DoD to VA care, following a permanent change of station [PCS]). Each RCC is located at a TBI clinical care center that is part of the DVBIC network of clinics and medical facilities specializing in TBI care—and serves a caseload drawn either from a defined geographic region of the country or from a specific military treatment facility (MTF). RCC services include education and support, referrals to local service providers, and systematic follow-up and tracking of TBI symptoms.

Purpose of the Report

This report summarizes the RAND Corporation's independent assessment of the structure, activities, and implementation of the DVBIC CCP. The assessment was conducted between April and July 2012. Although brief descriptions of the DVBIC CCP exist in the published literature, no thorough, complete, and publicly available description of the CCP is available. In addition to providing this description, the project sought to

1. document the history and implementation of the DVBIC CCP
2. identify target beneficiaries and document the reach of the program
3. explore perceived barriers to and facilitators of successful care coordination of TBI services
4. identify lessons CCP staff members have learned throughout the program's history, which may serve as a valuable resource to other care coordination programs.

Methods

To address the goals above, we conducted semistructured interviews in person with DVBIC CCP administrators and via telephone with RCCs between April 27, 2012, and July 12, 2012. These interviews included questions to prompt discussion of program services, history, eligibility criteria, population served, standards for delivery of program services, fidelity protocols, outreach activities, referral patterns, caseloads, RCC work environments, staffing structure, variation across offices, barriers and facilitators of successful care coordination, perceived program benefits, and opportunities for improvement. All interviews were conducted by a team of two qualitative interviewers and one research assistant and lasted 30 to 60 minutes.

At the time of the assessment, there were 14 RCCs. We received permission from program leadership to contact 12 of the 14. Of the 12 RCCs approached to complete interviews, 11 participated. In-person interviews were also conducted at CCP headquarters with the acting CCP program manager and the care coordinator liaison.

Finally, to assess CCP's web presence, we completed a content analysis of CCP websites, examining each CCP site's web materials for inclusion of the information necessary for a service member or veteran to determine the goals of the program, eligibility criteria, and self-referral process.

Innovative Practices

The CCP provides a unique bridge across systems of care and geographic regions for service members with a mild or moderate TBI that is symptomatic. Unlike care coordinators affiliated with a specific MTF, RCCs can follow patients as they transition from an inpatient facility to outpatient services, as they leave active duty and enter the VA system, and as they experience a PCS. These transitions are critical periods during which service members may drop out of services and may be especially challenging for those experiencing TBI. The RCC's proactive contacts with service members may help to ensure that service members with TBI in need of support services continue to receive them.

One important CCP role is to serve as a library of TBI-related resources nationwide. However, all RCCs are licensed nurses, social workers, or counselors, which allows them be more than a simple clearinghouse. They are able to provide direct services, such as supportive listening and encouragement. Their expertise in TBI, unique among care coordination programs, allows them to provide education to service members, veterans, and their families that is precisely targeted to their questions, concerns, and needs. Furthermore, their extensive knowledge of both TBI and support services nationwide is not limited to individuals eligible for program enrollment but is shared freely with anyone who calls the program.

Finally, the DVBIC CCP focuses on assisting individuals with mild TBI,[1] a population not served by other care coordination programs. Without the CCP, service members with mild TBI might "fall through the cracks" of the current military and VA health care system. The program has established strong collaborative ties with a handful of MTFs to ensure a regular, although declining, stream of patient referrals with diagnosed TBIs and unresolved symptoms. By proactively contacting identified service members, CCP serves a population that might not otherwise actively engage such services.

Recommendations

Despite many notable program strengths, several key issues were highlighted as potential challenges to program sustainability and/or expansion in the future. These included challenges related to (1) the flow of information throughout the CCP program, (2) a lack of clarity around core program features and standardization across sites relevant to these features, and (3) outreach. CCP staff consider outreach to referral organizations and to individuals who may benefit from the program both an essential feature of the program and critical to its sustainability. Yet interviewees almost universally cited this as the biggest challenge the program faces.

In 2011, the CCP caseload represented only 4.5 percent of the 24,883 service members diagnosed with TBI (DVBIC, 2012a). Although most cases of mild TBI resolve naturally, without interven-

---

[1]   A brain injury is classified as mild if the initial alteration and/or loss of consciousness lasts no longer than 24 hours and if motor and verbal responses remain relatively unimpaired immediately after the trauma.

tion, and would not need or benefit from CCP services, these data suggest that the CCP may not be reaching the full population of service members who would benefit from program services.

We recognize that the DVBIC CCP may not be able to implement all our recommendations, but we offer them for consideration because the CCP is continually being improved and refined. It is possible that involvement with an external evaluation, as well as recent changes in program leadership, may already have prompted program changes between the time of our assessment and the publication of this report. Therefore, our recommendations should be considered in light of any recent changes to the program.

Based on our assessment, we recommend the following changes to improve the flow of information across the CCP:

- Expand opportunities for RCCs to receive training that promotes their understanding of all systems of care (DoD, VA, and community).
- Facilitate uniform RCC access to relevant medical records and health information.
- Continue to develop centralized data and information sharing tools.

To improve CCP standardization, we recommend that the program do the following:

- Continue to address program variation across sites related to multiple lines of authority.
- Clarify core features of the program and assess the program's fidelity to them.
- Consider the value of the decentralized, regional system of RCC sites, as compared to a more centralized system.

To improve program outreach, we recommend that the CCP do the following:

- Clarify funding available to RCCs to promote outreach.
- Consider alternative staffing models to facilitate outreach.

- Develop clear, standardized program materials at the headquarters level that all RCCs can use in outreach efforts.
- Consider changing the program's name and the RCC job title to better align with program services and to reflect the focus on TBI.
- Create a uniform web presence that is easy to navigate.
- Leverage additional TBI screening data to identify service members who may benefit from program services.

Finally, we recommend conducting an **outcomes evaluation**. Ideally, an outcomes evaluation would compare the short- and long-term outcomes of individuals who received CCP services with the outcomes of individuals with unresolved TBI who did not receive program services. Such comparisons are critical for understanding the effectiveness of the CCP in improving the lives of service members with TBI.

Limitations

This scope of this assessment was limited. Given resource constraints, RAND did not conduct an outcomes evaluation and thus makes no claims about the effectiveness of program services or the utility of the program relative to other services. We did not speak to service members the program serves and did not collect data to document the outcomes of service members or veterans who participated in the program relative to those who had no access to program services. Instead, we intended to provide a publicly available document of the program's organization, services, and history; to summarize the program's promising and innovative practices; and to provide limited recommendations for program improvement. Given that the primary data source was interviews with program administrators and staff, this report largely reflects their perceptions of the program's strengths and limitations. To improve the evidence base for the program and to document the effectiveness or utility of the program, we recommend conducting an outcomes evaluation of the DVBIC CCP.

Conclusion

The DVBIC CCP is an attempt to bridge the gaps across systems of care for service members with TBIs. Analysis of this program identified innovative practices, continuing challenges, and lessons learned. The recommendations provided here suggest strategies for meeting these challenges while maintaining the benefits possible through this novel approach to care.

Acknowledgements

We gratefully acknowledge the assistance of Lori Dickerson-Odoms, M.P.C., Program Manager, Office of Care Coordination, and Kelley Wood, R.N., RCC Liaison, Care Coordinator Liaison at U.S. Army Network Enterprise Technology Command, as well as the DVBIC RCCs who provided invaluable input about the program. We also thank our colleagues Deborah Scharf, Rajeev Ramchand, Lisa Meredith, Mike Fisher, and Phyllis Gilmore for their careful reviews, valuable insights, and thoughtful comments on drafts of this report. In addition, we thank Anna Smith for the administrative support she provided preparing this document. We also thank our project monitor at the Defense Centers of Excellence for Psychological Health and Traumatic Brain Injury, Col Christopher Robinson, and CPT Dayami Liebenguth, Yonatan Tyberg, and Richard Sechrest for their support of our work.

Abbreviations

AHLTA   Armed Forces Health Longitudinal Technology Application

CCP   Care Coordination Program

DCoE   Defense Centers of Excellence for Psychological Health and Traumatic Brain Injury

DoD   Department of Defense

DVBIC   Defense and Veterans Brain Injury Center

IRG   Independent Review Group on Rehabilitative Care and Administrative Processes at Walter Reed Army Medical Center and National Naval Medical Center

LRMC   Landstuhl Regional Medical Center

MTF   military treatment facility

OEF   Operation Enduring Freedom

OIF   Operation Iraqi Freedom

RCC   regional care coordinator

REC   regional education coordinator

PCS   permanent change of station

TBI   traumatic brain injury

VA   Department of Veterans Affairs

CHAPTER ONE

Introduction

Between 2001 and 2011, 2.2 million service members were deployed in support of Operation Enduring Freedom (OEF) and Operation Iraqi Freedom (OIF) (Sayer, 2011). In the era of the all-volunteer force, the pace and demands of these conflicts have led to longer and more frequent deployments and historically high levels of participation by reserve forces (Hosek, Kavanagh and Miller, 2006; Chu, Speakes, and Gardner, 2007). Improvised explosive devices have been used extensively against U.S. forces during these conflicts and have been one of the leading causes of death. Injuries among those who survive an improvised explosive device blast often include traumatic brain injuries (TBIs), which have been called the signature injury of the OEF/OIF conflict (Riccitiello, 2006). This report focuses on TBIs among service members and one program to improve care for service members and veterans experiencing continued negative sequelae from a brain injury, the Defense and Veterans Brain Injury Center (DVBIC) Care Coordination Program (CCP).

Epidemiology of TBI

The annual number of active duty service members diagnosed with a TBI by a medical professional grew from 12,470 in 2002 to 32,001 in 2011 (DVBIC, 2012b). Although these frequencies account for all diagnosed TBIs, including non–combat related injuries, it is likely that most of the 2.6-fold increase over the past decade is attributable to OEF/OIF injuries.

The rate of diagnosed TBIs likely underestimates the true prevalence because many service members do not seek or receive medical services for their injuries. Population-level surveys of service members provide additional data and estimates of TBI that do not rely on individuals having sought services. In one study, 15 percent of Army soldiers indicated that, during their last OIF deployment, they had experienced a physical trauma accompanied by a loss of consciousness or altered mental state, which is a common marker of TBI (Hoge et al., 2008). A RAND Corporation study of 1,938 previously OEF/OIF-deployed service members estimated the prevalence of TBI to be between 16.4 and 22.7 percent among this group (95-percent confidence interval; Schell and Marshall, 2008). Members of the Army or Marine Corps, men, enlisted personnel, and younger service members are more likely than others to report a TBI during deployment (Schell and Marshall, 2008). Note, however, that these demographic variables are correlated with combat trauma exposures, which fully account for all group differences (Schell and Marshall, 2008).

Severity, Symptoms, and Clinical Course of TBI

The severity of a TBI is graded according to the nature of the trauma and the immediate symptoms. A mild TBI, also known as a concussion, is diagnosed if alterations in consciousness last no longer than 24 hours; there is either no loss of consciousness or a loss of consciousness that lasts no longer than 30 minutes; there is either no amnesia or amnesia that resolves in less than 24 hours; and motor, verbal, and eye-opening responses remain relatively unimpaired immediately following the trauma (American Congress of Rehabilitation Medicine, 1993; Department of Veterans Affairs [VA], 2010; Teasdale et al., 1979). Moderate and severe TBIs are marked by an altered mental state extending days or weeks; amnesia lasting longer than 24 hours; a loss of consciousness longer than 30 minutes; and impaired motor, verbal, and eye-opening responses immediately following the trauma. Among service members diagnosed with a TBI in 2011, approximately 77 percent were classified as mild (DVBIC, 2012b).

TBI symptoms vary significantly depending on the brain regions the trauma has affected. Most patients with TBI will experience some, but rarely all, of the following common symptoms: headache, confusion, agitation, slurred speech, fatigue, sleep disturbances, vestibular disturbances, weakness, sensory problems, memory and concentration difficulties, problems with judgment and executive control, mood changes, irritability, impulsivity, aggression, vomiting or nausea, and convulsions or seizures (VA, 2010; Helmick et al., 2006; McCrea et al., 2009). It is important to note that the severity rating of a TBI is determined by the severity of the symptoms arising immediately after the trauma and *not* to the severity of ongoing symptoms (VA, 2010; Helmick et al., 2006; McCrea et al., 2009). Thus, some service members with mild TBIs may experience persistent and debilitating symptoms, while some with moderate TBIs may recover quickly and fully. Note as well that the severity diagnosis is not updated over time. A moderate TBI is not reclassified as mild as symptoms resolve but rather retains the original classification as moderate.

Symptoms associated with mild TBI are typically temporary (Carroll et al., 2004). Eighty-five to 95 percent of civilian patients with a mild TBI can expect a full recovery, very often within one to two weeks of the trauma (Carroll et al., 2004; McCrea et al., 2009; Ruff, 2005). For military service members who screen positive for a mild TBI, 85 to 90 percent recover within three months (VA, 2010). Without appropriate medical and psychosocial support, the remaining 10 to 15 percent may experience difficulty with occupational, family, and social reintegration; may have depression and anxiety; or may isolate themselves from family and friends (VA, 2010). The degree of recovery from moderate and severe TBIs is highly variable and unpredictable. Some patients return to baseline functioning rapidly, while others must learn strategies to adjust to permanent changes in functioning (VA, 2010).

Cognitive Challenges Related to TBI Highlight Need for Care Coordination

TBI symptoms include a number of signature cognitive problems, such as difficulty concentrating, difficulty organizing thoughts, impaired executive functioning, and memory lapses. Unfortunately, these are the very capacities necessary to navigate a complex system of care. Many service members who experience a TBI must also cope with other injuries, such as bone fractures, amputations, burns, and spinal cord injuries, as a result of the precipitating blast or impact. In addition, such traumas may lead to or be concurrent with subsequent psychological health challenges, such as posttraumatic stress disorder and depression (Hoge et al., 2008). To receive adequate coverage for all their physical and psychological health needs, service members must coordinate necessary medical, psychological, neuropsychological, physical therapy, occupational therapy, and vocational services, among others. This task is difficult even for those without cognitive challenges and may prove overwhelming or impossible for those recovering from a TBI. Although a range of case management and care coordination supports is available in both the Department of Defense (DoD) and VA health systems to assist injured service members and veterans with such activities, none had focused exclusively on TBI prior to the establishment of the DVBIC CCP. In 2007, two reports were published highlighting concerns around the coordination of these supports as service members transitioned across systems of care.

In *Rebuilding the Trust,* the DoD Independent Review Group (IRG) on Rehabilitative Care and Administrative Processes at Walter Reed Army Medical Center and National Naval Medical Center evaluated the rehabilitative care and administrative processes at Walter Reed Army Medical Center (IRG, 2007) following a *Washington Post* article on poor conditions (Priest and Hull, 2007). Deficits in the continuum of care were identified as one of the primary problems in the system (IRG, 2007). The report noted that, despite the best efforts of DVBIC, care for TBI was "neither coordinated nor consistent" (IRG, 2007, p. 17). The IRG report also broadly noted a systematic breakdown in the transition between DoD and the VA as injured service members transition to veteran status. Finally, the review group recognized the unfair burden placed on family members to navigate a complex system on behalf of their service members without adequate support.

A report from the President's Commission on Care for America's Returning Warriors (2007) focused on military-to-civilian transitions among returning OEF/OIF wounded service members and the coordination of key health, employment, and other benefits and services. In this report, commission members recommended establishing a network of highly skilled recovery coordinators to serve as a single point of contact for service members and be responsible for ensuring the execution of each wounded service member's recovery plan. The commission noted that family support is critical and recommended expanding coverage of respite care, providing caregiver training, and expanding the Family Medical Leave Act. The recommended system of federal recovery coordinators has been successfully implemented, and service members with moderate or severe TBIs now have comprehensive recovery plans and a recovery coordinator to manage implementation of those plans. Note, however, that service members with mild TBIs typically are not served by federal recovery coordinators.

DVBIC Care Coordination Program

In 2007, in response to many of the concerns that the above two reports raised, DVBIC launched the regional CCP to provide services to active duty service members, veterans, and current or former National Guard members and Reservists with ongoing symptoms associated with a mild or moderate TBI incurred while serving in OEF/OIF.[1] DVBIC is the DoD-supported, operational component of the Defense Centers of Excellence for Psychological Health and Traumatic Brain Injury (DCoE) that specializes in TBI. It has provided such services as population-level TBI screening, health care provider training, and direct support to service members affected by a TBI since 1992.

---

[1]   Hereafter, the term *service member* will be used to refer to active duty service members, veterans, and current or former National Guard and Reservists.

DVBIC viewed the CCP as a natural extension of its ongoing work to support service members with TBI through clinical, research, and educational programs. DVBIC leadership felt such a program could be readily implemented given its existing national network of clinical care sites. Regional care coordinators (RCCs) were hired, trained, and tasked with ensuring that service members remain connected to necessary services, particularly during difficult transition points (e.g., during the transition from DoD to VA care, following a permanent change of station [PCS]). Each RCC is located at one of DVBIC's clinical care centers and serves a caseload drawn either from a defined geographic region or from a specific military treatment facility (MTF) that specializes in treating TBI.

The services RCCs provide have three primary components. First, RCCs provide **education and support** to service members with TBIs and their family members. They provide information about TBI, including common and less-typical symptoms, types of treatment, and the variation in time courses toward recovery. Importantly, this educational component is individualized to the unique needs of a given service member and is provided on an as-needed basis, as service members and their families have concerns and questions. RCCs also provide a "listening ear" to support service members who may be frustrated, angry, confused, or depressed about their injuries.

Second, RCCs provide **recommendations for local or community services** that are matched to the service members' needs. These recommendations are not formal referrals (i.e., clinician-to-clinician referral for a patient to see a specialist). Rather, RCCs serve as a clearinghouse of all TBI services available to service members in their region. After assessing the service member and his or her needs, an RCC will recommend that he or she contact a program(s) in his or her vicinity that can provide services matched to his or her unique needs. RCCs provide the service member with a description of the local program's services and the information he or she needs to initiate contact with the program (e.g., telephone, address, point of contact). After providing the recommendation, RCCs typically do not contact the program to share clinical information about the service member and do not schedule the appointment or tell the program to be expecting a call from the service member. The CCP's philosophical goal is to foster self-reliance by leaving these tasks in the hands of the service member or family member. However, RCCs may call the service member to confirm that he or she was able to reach the program and make an appointment or to help problem-solve if the service member was unsuccessful.

Finally, RCCs complete regular **check-in calls to track TBI symptoms and recovery.** These calls are scheduled for three, six, nine, 12, 18, and 24 months after a service member enters the program. During each call, symptoms are assessed with the CCP Checklist, which includes 28 domains (e.g., headaches, sleep, memory, depression, relationship problems). Domains cover physical symptoms, cognitive difficulties, psychological health issues, and psychosocial problems. Each domain is coded as symptom present or absent, and when a symptom is present, RCCs document the details. The checklist was developed by the program and relies on self-reporting by the service member. Data from these checklists are maintained in a spreadsheet, which allows RCCs to monitor client symptoms as they resolve and to identify new symptoms in a timely manner. Although much of the work of an RCC is to provide education about medical symptoms and recommendations to manage them, RCCs also provide assistance as the symptoms resolve in addressing nonmedical needs, such as work reintegration, social or relationship conflict, or continuing education.

To be eligible for program services, a service member must have served during the Gulf War, OEF/OIF, or the Global War on Terror and have a documented diagnosis of TBI that has not yet resolved. The majority of CCP referrals come from Landstuhl Regional Medical Center (LRMC) in Germany. Service members who experience a traumatic injury in theater receive initial medical attention and screening at LRMC. While there, all patients undergo extensive neurocognitive testing to evaluate possible TBI. LRMC then forwards to the CCP the names, contact information, and location on redeployment of all service members who screen positive for a mild or moderate TBI and require services. CCP leadership then distributes the information to the RCC serving the returning service member's region, and the RCC contacts the service member directly. Program referrals are also received from MTFs and VA providers, and individuals may also self-refer.

Assessment of the DVBIC Care Coordination Program

Although brief descriptions of the DVBIC CCP exist in the published literature (French, Parkinson, and Massetti, 2011; Jaffee et al., 2009), no thorough, complete, and publicly available description of the CCP is available. Therefore, this project sought to

1. document the history and implementation of the DVBIC CCP
2. identify target beneficiaries and document the reach of the program
3. explore perceived barriers and facilitators to successful care coordination of TBI services
4. identify lessons learned by the CCP staff throughout the program's history, which may serve as a valuable resource to other care coordination programs.

Given the time and resource constraints of this project, RAND did not conduct an outcomes evaluation and thus makes no claims about the effectiveness of program services or the utility of the program relative to other services.

Methodology

We conducted semistructured interviews with DVBIC CCP administrators and RCCs between April 27 and July 12, 2012. These interviews included questions to prompt discussion of program services, history, eligibility criteria, population served, standards for delivery of program services, fidelity protocols, outreach activities, referral patterns, caseloads, RCC work environments, staffing structure, variation across offices, barriers and facilitators of successful care coordination, perceived program benefits, and opportunities for improvement. All interviews were conducted by a rotating team of two (out of three) qualitative interviewers and one research assistant (who took notes). Each interviewer participated in roughly two-thirds of the interviews, which improved standardization across interviews.

At the time of the assessment, there were 14 RCCs. We received permission from program leadership to contact 12 of the 14. Of the

12 RCCs approached to complete interviews, 11 participated. We also conducted in-person interviews at CCP headquarters with the acting CCP program manager and the RCC liaison.[2] Interviews with RCCs lasted 30 to 60 minutes, and the interview with program administrators lasted three hours; the team research assistant took notes during interviews. After all interviews were complete, we conducted a thematic analysis of interview notes.

Finally, the team completed a content analysis of DVBIC CCP websites. Methodology for the web content analysis is summarized in Chapter Five, with additional details provided in Appendix A.

Organization of This Report

This report documents the DVBIC CCP's history and services, summarizes lessons learned about barriers to and facilitators of TBI care coordination, and provides recommendations for future research and potential program improvements. Chapter Two describes the administrative and staffing structure of the program, including the decentralized model for the program. Chapter Three describes the characteristics of current RCCs, their tasks, caseloads, and training opportunities. In Chapter Four, we review program eligibility criteria, the current population served, and opportunities to expand the reach of the program. Chapter Five focuses on outreach to eligible service members and treatment facilities, marketing, and branding issues. Throughout the report, we summarize the innovative components of the program, including the unique emphasis on mild TBI, proactive recruitment of eligible service members, and the crucial bridge provided by RCCs across systems of care and during periods of transition. Chapter Six describes potential recommendations to overcome program challenges.

---

[2] It should be noted that, at the time of this assessment, the CCP program was undergoing a change in leadership.

CHAPTER TWO

Structure and Infrastructure of the DVBIC Care Coordination Program

This chapter provides an overview of the program structure, staffing, and administrative lines of authority. CCP's decentralized nature has advantages but also creates challenges, as RCCs both report to CCP headquarters and reside in a local facility. In this chapter, we outline the implications of these program characteristics, highlighting innovative practices and lessons learned.

Program Structure

As noted above, DVBIC is the operational component of DCoE that provides such services as population-level TBI screening, health care provider training, and direct support to service members and veterans affected by TBIs. DVBIC headquarters are located in Washington, D.C., and there are 17 care and treatment sites, including one in Landstuhl, Germany, to provide reasonably accessible services to service members and veterans across the country.

CCP is a DVBIC program that operates within its geographically decentralized system. Each DVBIC site provides care to service members residing in the region; similarly, the CCP offices located at each site coordinate care for the same service members. RCCs are located at 13 of the 17 DVBIC treatment sites. The remaining DVBIC sites do not currently have RCCs (VA Boston Healthcare System, Camp Pendleton, Fort Belvoir Community Hospital, LRMC).[1] Of the 14 RCCs, eight work in offices at military medical centers, four work at VA hospitals, and two work at civilian partner sites. Typically, there is one RCC per site; however, in one high-caseload site (Fort Carson, Colorado), two RCCs share the duties.

CCP has two types of care coordinators: (1) *Nonembedded* RCCs are assigned a geographical region of four to ten states and serve all eligible service members or veterans residing in the region, and (2) *embedded* RCCs serve a single MTF and coordinate care only for service members who are receiving or have received care at the affiliated treatment facility. Ten of the 14 care coordinators are nonembedded RCCs, and the remaining four are embedded RCCs. However, all care coordinators are referred to as RCCs, regardless of whether or not they are embedded. The map in Figure 2.1 shows RCC regions and the location of each RCC office.

Staffing Structure and Lines of Authority

CCP administrators, located at DVBIC Headquarters, support 14 RCCs, affiliated with the DBVIC sites nationwide. The program manager is responsible for program infrastructure, maintaining standard operating procedures, and administrative coordination between the CCP, DVBIC, DCoE, and site leadership at each of the CCP offices. The program manager is also responsible for the CCP database, which records RCC caseloads, referral patterns, and rates of follow-up. The RCC liaison is responsible for all tasks related to supervision of RCCs and clinical services. He or she chairs biweekly teleconferences, provides as-needed clinical supervision, coordinates access to electronic medical records for RCCs without access, and evaluates the performance of each RCC annually.

---

[1] These numbers were current at the time of data collection (April 27–July 12, 2012), although program leadership was considering adding RCCs at LRMC and the National Intrepid Center of Excellence (which would be the first RCC at a non-DVBIC site).

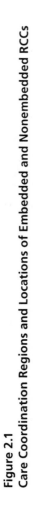

Figure 2.1
Care Coordination Regions and Locations of Embedded and Nonembedded RCCs

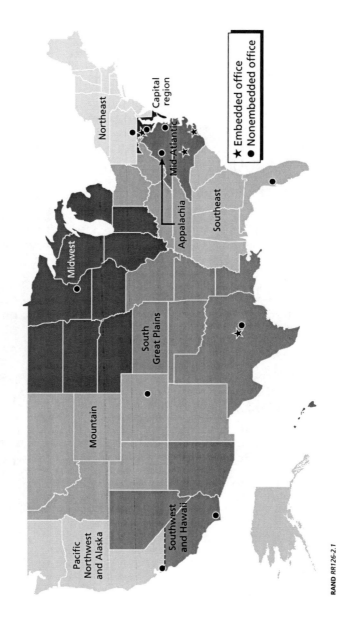

RAND *RR1126-2.1*

RCCs are CCP staff located at DVBIC sites; thus, RCCs answer to multiple lines of authority. Program administration (e.g., coordinating referrals from Landstuhl, training, performance reviews) comes from CCP headquarters, but day-to-day operation is often managed by the administrators of the local DVBIC site. As discussed below, where centralized authority ends and local authority begins is not always clear and appears to vary based on site characteristics. Although RCCs and CCP administrators note that multiple lines of authority can be challenging at times, these relationships also provide multiple avenues for resources for RCCs (e.g., funds, information, training). Figure 2.2 characterizes these relationships and the links among the RCCs and community providers.

To better understand the implications of the CCP structure and lines of authority, part of our conversations with RCCs centered on organizational characteristics. Specifically, conversations included the following topics:

- relationships with CCP headquarters and the local site
- the flow of information, both to and from CCP headquarters and among RCCs
- referrals within and between regions
- data tracking
- performance evaluation
- lines of authority.

In these and other parts of our discussions, several themes arose, which centered on these unique organizational characteristics. Each of these themes is described below.

Relationship with CCP Headquarters and RCCs

The RCCs indicated that CCP headquarters acts as a central information clearinghouse, but RCCs ranged widely in the extent to which they used this resource. In particular, the RCCs noted that headquarters acts as the conduit for referrals from LRMC, provides initial

Figure 2.2
Lines of Authority and Lines of Resources for RCCs

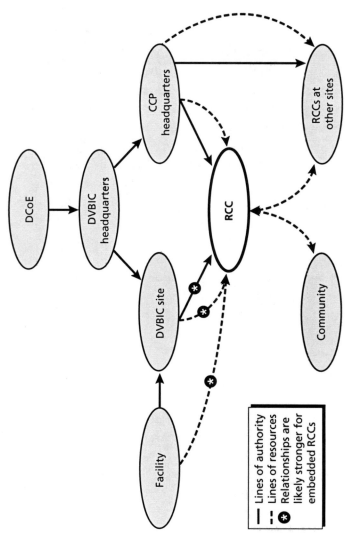

RAND RR126-2.2

training to recent hires, runs biweekly teleconferences, collects weekly reports of RCC activities for tracking purposes, and conducts annual performance reviews. RCCs attend biweekly education and supervision teleconferences with headquarters leadership. They described the leadership as an accessible resource to be used as needed. Generally, the relationship was described positively, although RCC descriptions of the role of headquarters in day-to-day operations varied, ranging from regular consultations to relatively infrequent interactions. It is unclear whether this variability is due to differential needs across RCCs or to recent changes in leadership at headquarters.

In general, management from CCP headquarters appears to give RCCs a good deal of independence, and with the exception of required reporting (e.g., suicidality) and biweekly teleconferences, clinical supervision is provided on an as-needed basis. RCCs described acting fairly independently of headquarters in most day-to-day operations. In many ways, this appears necessary, as each RCC reacts to the realities in his or her site and region, and in many cases, RCCs more appropriately deal directly with each other. For example, one RCC noted that, when coordinating the transfer of care for individuals moving to another region of the country, she typically does not engage headquarters but rather works directly with the receiving RCC. These warm handoffs between RCCs were endorsed in several discussions. As highlighted by another RCC,

> It's hard to say what I do without talking about the larger care coordination network, as we do transfer between each other, which happens fairly often.

This mutual support among the RCCs extended to information sharing, advice, and clinical support. As one RCC noted, networking among the RCCs, and the associated ability to tap into resources around the nation, was one of the primary benefits of the DVBIC RCC program (see Figure 2.2).

That said, RCCs also noted that this information does not always flow as freely as it could. For example, RCCs currently manage their own databases of client information, including branch of service, rank, date of birth, symptoms at intake and over time, current and past treatments, and other issues, and this information is not systematically shared among RCCs. RCCs mentioned that the development of a shared client-tracking system has been discussed. However, such a system is not yet available. Implementing an information-sharing system could benefit the program by adding structure and systemization to communication and collaboration.

Integration with Local Facilities

Multiple RCCs noted the benefits of being physically and operationally integrated with their DVBIC clinical care site, including the ability to check in with current patients regularly and the ease of access to medical professionals, if necessary, for consultation or advice. In most instances, the RCCs are housed in or near the TBI clinic or with the DVBIC staff. Weekly site-team meetings, cooperation with DVBIC regional education coordinators (RECs),[2] and close relationships with TBI site coordinators can lead to identification with the local DVBIC site as much as, or more than, with the national CCP program. Depending on the degree of support and integration, this program structure can be viewed as an advantage or a challenge. One RCC noted, for example, that her local site was a valuable source of training and knowledge:

> I was blessed with my site, but others are out there without the internal support at the site.

For example, those who were less well integrated into their site indicated that they were sometimes perceived as outsiders and were not fully supported (even denied adequate working space on occasion). One avenue for facilitating integration may be to provide RCCs with

---

[2]   Duties of the DVBIC RCCs also vary by site but include educating families and service members about TBI; training hospital staff and health care providers on TBI and TBI-related topics; and reaching out to military facilities, VA facilities, and the community throughout the site's region to provide education on issues related to TBI.

training to familiarize them with the organization and the organizational culture of the facility in which they are embedded.

Centralization Versus Decentralization of CCP Service Delivery

The pros and cons of the program's current structure make determining the optimal balance of centralization and decentralization a challenge. On the one hand, there are advantages to a decentralized system, in which RCCs are distributed around the country and operating relatively independently (as opposed to being centrally located and, for example, using a central telephone bank). Indeed, there is some indication that the system may not be sufficiently decentralized to fully support the entire population eligible for program services. For instance, many nonembedded RCCs indicated that, despite being responsible for multistate regions, the majority of their caseloads are drawn from the local facility and surrounding area. Although DVBIC sites were selected strategically to reflect concentrations of returning service members, RCCs repeatedly mentioned that a unique benefit of the RCC program is the ability to help individuals who have recently separated from the military and may be struggling with how to find and access resources in a community setting. It is this population that the existing program structure may currently be underserving. Furthermore, several RCCs noted that Guard and Reserve members are particularly challenging to reach because they quickly reintegrate into their home communities. Although no data were obtained on the geographic locations of individuals utilizing RCC services, our interviews with RCCs suggested that individuals more proximal to the location of the RCC are more likely to be involved with the program than are those who reside further away but still within the RCC's region (e.g., in a neighboring state).

On the other hand, although many benefits of a decentralized system were noted, both administrators and RCCs saw value in centralization in other domains. Since nonembedded RCCs conduct almost all program correspondence by telephone, they need not be physically located within their respective regions. They noted that a central "bank" of RCCs would allow them to work together in the same office building with colleagues and administrative support. Despite noting that, under the current system, colleagues were only "a phone call away," several RCCs still saw colocation as increasing the ease and likelihood of brief consultations with one another. One disadvantage of a centralized office for all RCCs would be that outreach to other MTFs, VA hospitals, and treatment facilities in the RCC's region would be more difficult. However, this limitation applies to a decentralized system as well because, even in the current system, RCCs often voiced a desire for more travel resources.

RCCs Face Varied Lines of Authority

As illustrated in Figure 2.2, RCCs face multiple lines of authority, both through CCP headquarters and the local DVBIC site. For example, RCC performance evaluations include input not only from headquarters but also from the local program manager, who may have more day-to-day oversight over the RCC, even if that oversight is informal. As with other aspects of the program, the relative dominance of different authorities appeared to vary across sites. One RCC noted that,

> We have duties that are site specific, so we answer to our sites, as well as headquarters.

Another RCC noted that headquarters officially supervises the RCCs but that her site director is more involved in day-to-day operations (including clinical supervision). In contrast, another RCC stated that her primary contacts were with headquarters rather than with local management. As one RCC described, "I treat it like I have two or three bosses." This same RCC went on to describe the confusion that this can cause:

> It seemed at times that the sites may not have communicated with headquarters, and it was put back on me to be the middle man to communicate, and that was very frustrating.

The role of local management, therefore, ranged from acting as a primary boss to simply requiring updates as a professional courtesy.

DVBIC appears to be addressing this variation and the resulting uncertainty. As noted by one RCC,

> I have seen a change recently. It seems like there is more of a direc-
> tive to go through headquarters on certain things and through
> sites for certain things. At least more clarity on who we go to on
> certain things.

Another RCC reported that the local program manager originally functioned as the primary manager but now serves a more administrative function, with CCP headquarters taking on more of a clinical management role.

Access to Medical Records

One difference among RCCs is the type of facility in which they are housed—military, VA, or community partner. Generally speaking, RCCs at MTFs reported ready access to military medical records through the Armed Forces Health Longitudinal Technology Application (AHLTA), and as one MTF-located RCC stated, "having access to medical records is very helpful—almost necessary." Another pointed out that,

> I can tell where patients have gone, if they've been readmitted,
> find new contact information, do chart reviews—it really helps.

In contrast, RCCs at VA sites typically only have direct access to the medical records of patients seen at that particular VA facility, and community-based RCCs have no direct access to medical records. Given that details of the injury and initial treatment records typically reside in the military health system, VA- and community-based RCCs rely on patient interviews for gaining necessary information. As one RCC noted,

> I'm at a VA. I have access to records of people who come to my VA only. I don't have access to AHLTA or other VA records. Other RCCs use AHLTA to give them a sense of what's going on with a service member. I have to go off of self-report.

Another VA-based RCC said,

> I have had challenges where I needed to follow a service member and don't have anything more current about whether they are getting care.

A third VA-based RCC noted that,

> [Having access to medical records] would make my job a bit more well rounded . . . since I won't be blindsided.

Although not all RCCs have access to medical records, RCCs can ask the individual for permission to talk to his or her case manager about information that would help the RCC identify appropriate resources. As noted above, RCCs reported that the development of a sharable CCP database of clients has been discussed. Unfortunately, such a database has yet to be established and, to date, remains an unmet need.

Institutional Knowledge Tends to Be System Specific

As an RCC at a VA location noted, if you are working with the military but are not affiliated with a military site, it can be difficult to know who to contact and how to structure the contact: "You have to have a little finesse." When asked about additional training, another VA-based RCC noted that it would be helpful to receive specific training on the military health system:

> The military piece. What's going on with the process from start to finish with the service members who are coming through, what's going on with their injuries, how they are triaged. I'd love to go to Landstuhl [LRMC]. I think probably the coordinators located

in the MTFs would feel the same way about wanting to learn more about the VAs. That's where the strongest barrier is between the DoD side and the civilian and VA systems. It sets up a line between the coordinators.

These boundaries between MTF, VA-, and civilian-based RCCs represent a notable limitation of the program, given that one of the primary aims of the program, as noted by the RCCs, is "filling in the cracks" between the military, VA, and civilian systems and, accordingly, catching individuals who might otherwise "fall through the cracks." This language was commonly used by RCCs, suggesting that the program's role as a safety net is part of its core identity. And while the ability to bridge the gap between systems is indeed a program focus and one of the program's strengths, this strength does not seem to reach its full potential because of the program's own gaps—between DVBIC sites with different affiliations. However, it is important to note that this challenge is not unique to the CCP program, and other programs focused on bridging gaps between health care systems likely also face it.

Innovative Practices and Lessons Learned

RCCs bridge systems of care and geographic regions. Unlike care coordinators affiliated with a specific MTF, an RCC can follow a patient as he or she transitions from an inpatient facility to outpatient services, as he or she leaves active duty and enters the VA system, or during and after a PCS. These transitions are critical periods in which service members with TBI may drop out of services. To the extent that individuals still need the support, RCCs can ensure that service members with TBI secure appropriate care in a new location or from a new care provider.

Decentralization has advantages. Being located in communities around the country, RCCs are closer to their caseloads and are able to reach out to and develop expertise on their regions more easily than under a centralized system.

Balancing multiple lines of authority can be challenging. CCP is a national program that houses its representatives within an existing regional site. Therefore, a balance must be struck between at least two lines of authority. This appears to have been a challenge for the program, as it likely would be for any such program. Recent efforts to clarify these relationships appear to be addressing some of the challenges.

Sharing information across military, VA, and community systems remains a challenge. It is likely that gap-bridging programs for other service member populations would face similar challenges.

CHAPTER THREE

Regional Care Coordinators

Given CCP's decentralized administrative structure, most RCCs must be able to work independently and, in some ways, run their own "offices." Administrators at CCP headquarters note that they explicitly hire for this trait and also expect and encourage independent functioning. Perhaps in part due to this requirement, the program hires a cadre of highly skilled and educated care coordinators. Other case management programs may rely on bachelors-level staff, but CCP recruits licensed clinicians. Thus, the RCCs themselves are one of the unique and innovative components of the program.

RCC Education and Experience

Each RCC is a licensed nurse or has a masters-level education in social work or counseling psychology. All RCCs have either a license to practice independently within their specialty area or a Certified Brain Injury Specialist certificate. Although RCCs do not provide diagnostic or medical advice or services, they are required to be aware of the broad range of experiences that a service member with a TBI may face and to be knowledgeable about the systems of care he or she may need to access. Therefore, CCP makes it an explicit requirement that care coordinators have advanced clinical degrees. CCP administrators state that successful care coordinators are able to work without daily supervision. For example,

I'm looking for someone who is a real go-getter. On a day-to-day basis, [management] is just not there. They have to show real initiative and be confident in what they're doing.

RCCs manage their caseloads, clinical tasks, and outreach responsibilities relatively independently and have the authority to individualize their care coordination approaches to meet the needs of their unique caseloads and the systems of care with which they interact.

In 2012, the median caseload RCCs (n = 11) reported in our sample was 70, with a range of 36 to 127 cases. Caseloads were reported as the number of cases the RCC was following at the time of the interview. Median RCC tenure was two years and ranged from seven months to three years and seven months. See Table 3.1 for additional RCC characteristics.

Table 3.1
Findings from the Assessment Characteristics of Regional Care Coordinators and Offices

	n	Percent	Median	Range
Caseload[a]			70	36–127
Tenure with CCP (years)[a]			2	0.6–3.6
Experience (years)[a]				
Case management or care coordination			5	0.6–17
Working with people with a TBI			5	0.6–22.5
Working with service members or veterans			3.6	0.6–15
RCC type				
Embedded	4	29		
Nonembedded	10	71		
RCC office location				
VA health care system	4	29		
MTF	8	57		
Civilian treatment center	2	14		

[a] Self-reported data (n = 11) missing for three RCCs who did not complete semistructured interviews.

RCC Training

Training for RCCs has evolved considerably since program inception. RCCs hired soon after program implementation reported limited or no formal training and reported feeling "thrown into it." However, program administrators stated that there has been increased attention to training as the program has evolved and matured. Currently, when a new care coordinator begins his or her position with the DVBIC, an effort is made to have the previous person in the position provide on-the-job training to smooth the transition between the departing and newly hired RCCs, although this is not always possible, depending on when the new RCC is hired. In addition, new RCCs travel to visit CCP headquarters and receive training on standard operating procedures, learn about the CCP tracking database, and learn how to submit weekly reports about their cases and the services provided. New hires also work closely with the RCC liaison to learn about the range of clinical needs of service members in the program, to learn strategies for maintaining community contacts and referrals, and to practice typical interactions with service members. In some cases, new RCCs received travel support to visit other sites, where they shadowed and learned from more-senior care coordinators. Several RCCs noted that it was helpful to train with these RCCs at locations other than their own.

All RCCs are licensed in their specialty areas and are granted work hours to complete necessary continuing education credits to maintain their licenses. Care coordinators also report that they receive continued informal training and clinical supervision during twice-monthly teleconferences between CCP headquarters and all RCCs and that they take advantage of relevant talks and seminars at their respective MTF or VA locations. Finally, as part of outreach activities, some RCCs travel to TBI-relevant conferences to give presentations or staff booths providing information about the DVBIC CCP. During their visits to these conferences, many also attend relevant talks and training sessions.

Recently hired care coordinators typically reported being satisfied with training opportunities:

I think they did a good job training me . . . . In this line of work, each case is not always the same. . . . Learning about resources available takes time, . . . but I think I was trained appropriately.

Others added that it is impossible to ever be "fully trained" on TBI and that "I think we'd all love to have more training. . . . I really don't think we'll ever know everything we need to know."

Workload and Typical Tasks of RCCs

RCCs engage in three primary activities: clinical tasks, identification of local support services, and development of a referral network.

Clinical Tasks

The primary RCC responsibilities are to coordinate the care of each client in his or her caseload and to provide support and referrals to others who contact the program but do not become official cases. RCCs estimate that they spend 50 to 80 percent of their time engaged in these types of clinical tasks during a typical workweek.

Assessing Client Needs

RCCs report that most of the time invested in a case occurs when a service member first enters the program. The RCC will conduct a 30- to 60-minute intake to assess all the participant's needs. In some cases, when needs are limited, the RCC may be able to provide all necessary recommendations during the first contact. For other cases, he or she may spend a few days to a few weeks placing calls to various providers and facilities to locate appropriate recommendations in the service member's immediate community or at nearby facilities. If the RCC has access to AHLTA medical records, he or she may also invest time in learning more about the service member's initial injury and subsequent treatment course. As initial recommendations are made, the RCC may place follow-up calls to the service member to confirm that they were able to schedule an appointment or, later, that they attended a scheduled appointment. One RCC noted:

I may contact them a couple of times a week, or once a month . . . ;
it depends on their needs. If they're going to their first appointment at the VA on Wednesday, I'm calling them on Thursday to
see how it went, and if there's anything else I can do for them.

The RCC may also assess whether the service member was satisfied with his or her care and may provide additional recommendations
until he or she feels the service member or veteran has a stable network
of care providers, at which point, the frequency of contact declines.
Individuals are encouraged to contact their RCCs as new needs arise.

Following Up with Clients

In addition to contacts the RCC initiates at will, the program also
dictates regularly scheduled follow-up calls for active cases to assess
the service member's recovery and to identify new needs, as evaluated
via the CCP Checklist. These calls are conducted three, six, nine, 12,
18, and 24 months after the initial intake. If new needs are identified during follow-up calls, the care coordinator will provide appropriate additional recommendations for services or providers. Note that
RCCs are not limited to contacting service members only at the official follow-up points and may use their discretion to check in with
service members at other high-needs times. For example, RCCs noted
that, at around 12 months following intake, service members may be
transitioning from active duty to veteran status and often benefit from
increased support and coordination services at that juncture.

Although follow-up calls officially continue for 24 months, data
we received from the Care Coordination Office reveals that the likelihood of successfully contacting a service member for a follow-up call
declines precipitously over time. In 2011, for a total caseload of 1,129,
RCCs completed 628 three-month calls, 379 six-month calls, 217 one-
year calls, and 91 two-year calls. RCCs explain that some of this drop-
off over time can be attributed to an inability to contact service members due to expired contact information. More often, however, service
members are not contacted for these late follow-ups because RCC have
already closed the cases.

Closing Cases

Cases are closed at RCC discretion, but the decision is typically made in consultation with the service member. One RCC told the interviewer that he or she closes a case when

> [The service member] tells me everything is going OK. They're getting all the services they need. I'll say, "do you want me to check back with you?" and if they say no, I'll give them my name [and] contact information, and I'll say to them, "I'm not going to be calling you, but feel free to call me back, let me know."

Most RCCs reported that their cases are reasonably stable within a year: "Most close out at six months." Similarly,

> A lot of them, I hang on to for three months, and then they're out. . . . It's very rare that I keep them to 24 months; by that time, they're well embedded. You do a lot of front loading, a lot of legwork in the beginning, and by the three-month mark, they're doing pretty good.

In future evaluation efforts, CCP might consider documenting the proportion of cases RCCs close before the final follow-up call or after the final follow-up call or that are lost to attrition. This information may allow program leadership to revisit program goals. For example, if nearly all cases are closed prior to 24 months, the program may wish to reconsider the purpose of official follow-up calls that do not, in fact, occur. If, on the other hand, regular and prolonged contact is considered a central component of the program, the program leadership may wish to reconsider allowing cases to be closed early.

Identifying Local Support Services

To recommend appropriate, well matched, and reasonably close service providers to clients residing in an RCC's four- to ten-state region, nonembedded RCCs must maintain an extensive database of TBI (and non-TBI) medical, psychological, and other providers. When the first RCCs started at the program, no such database existed, and a tremendous amount of manpower was required to build this resource. In

2012, RCCs reported having relatively mature databases of regional service providers, but these databases continuously evolve as services are added, disbanded, and changed. Each RCC is responsible for developing and managing his or her own database with services unique to the region. Even for stable treatment facilities, regular and expected staff turnover ensures that contact information must be continuously checked and updated. It does not appear that RCCs currently have the resources to judge systematically the quality of services from these providers. New resources in geographically distant areas are added as needed, for example, when an RCC adds a client residing in an area that has not yet been researched for the database. The task of maintaining a region's database and identifying relevant resources falls with each RCC and continues to be a significant component of the nonembedded RCC's workload.

Developing a Referral Network

Finally, RCCs are expected to maintain contacts with service providers and treatment facilities in their region that may be sources of referrals to the program. This outreach is designed to ensure that service providers who are responsible for service members with mild to moderate TBIs are aware of CCP and will refer eligible patients to the program. Several RCCs noted that updating their recommendation list and reaching out to a provider for referrals are often accomplished in the same contact.

RCC-Driven Variability Across Sites

Within the program, there seems to be some tension between encouraging RCCs to act independently to tailor their services to their regions' populations and efforts toward program standardization. In interviews with CCP headquarters staff, a program administrator stated that

> [CCP is a] standardized program with SOPs [standardized operating procedures] that direct how the follow-ups are conducted, what we're documenting. . . . There are some administrative dif-

ferences [across sites], but as far as the program, what we're doing, it's standardized.

However, in our interviews with RCCs, we noted considerable variation in the focus across offices. We suspect that some of this variation may be linked to the unique strengths and skills of each RCC and the site at which he or she is located. For example, some nurse RCCs seemed to focus on the detailed medical needs of patients. Other RCCs discussed additional occupational and social components associated with recovery from TBI. For example, one RCC discussed higher education at length, noting efforts to facilitate access to job retraining and college; other care coordinators never discussed educational needs. Some RCCs felt it was important to continue following cases, even after service members settle into stable, local support services to be available when service members experience the disruption of a PCS or a transition out of the service. Others took the approach of closing cases as soon as service members state they have no further needs. Although this evaluation included no formal assessment of the services CCP clients received, discussions with care coordinators suggest that a service member residing in one geographic area (served by a particular RCC) may receive slightly different services with a slightly different focus and length of follow-up from a service member assigned to another RCC. The precise range of this variability is uncertain and may warrant further study if program administration feels that program fidelity is an important goal.

Innovative Practices and Lessons Learned

The CCP employs licensed, clinically skilled care coordinators. All RCCs are clinically trained and licensed, which allows them to be more than a clearinghouse of TBI resources. They are able to provide important, direct services. For example, many care coordinators noted that sometimes a service member's greatest need was for a "listening ear," someone who would provide support and a place to vent his or her frustration, fear, concerns, and grief. All RCCs were well prepared to play this important role.

RCCs possess unique, TBI-specific expertise. RCCs' unique expertise in TBI allows them to provide education to service members and their families that is precisely targeted to their questions, concerns, and needs. This focus on TBI differentiates it from other such programs.

Regular and proactive RCC follow-up calls are a program asset. Regularly scheduled follow-up calls, when they occur, provide an opportunity to discover new needs that have surfaced since the last contact. Although service members may develop new concerns, questions, or needs between contacts (e.g., their treating physicians retire, they decide to return to school), they may not proactively contact their RCCs for assistance. The regularly scheduled follow-up calls provide a strategy for catching these needs that may otherwise go unnoticed.

Job training continues to evolve. Given the unique role RCCs fill, no newly hired RCC is likely to have perfectly matched experience in care coordination for service members with TBI. Since 2007, the program has expanded and formalized the support and training that new RCCs receive, and this effort appears to have been successful, with recent hires reporting satisfaction with the training they received.

CHAPTER FOUR

Program Eligibility and Population Served

This chapter provides detail on the eligibility criteria for CCP services and the population served. It also describes the referral process and how individuals become engaged with the program. These criteria, target populations, and referral sources were developed at the height of the OEF/OIF, with an eye toward ensuring that those most likely to benefit from program services were identified and engaged. However, given the changing landscape of U.S. military involvement overseas and the impending drawdown of troops, the previously defined criteria and approaches to identifying eligible populations are beginning to introduce a variety of challenges that may threaten program sustainability. In this chapter, we outline these challenges and recommend that CCP begin to plan strategically for continued relevance in the future.

Eligibility for CCP Services

RCCs serve two primary populations. The first includes individuals who are eligible for the program and who are added to an RCC's official caseload. To be eligible for program services, individuals must be active duty service members or veterans of the Gulf War, OEF/OIF, or the Global War on Terror, including Guard and Reserve members, with a documented diagnosis of TBI that has not yet resolved. Both the RCC and the service member must agree that continued contact, monitoring, and care coordination would be helpful.

RCCs also serve a second, heterogeneous group of individuals who do not meet the official eligibility criteria. This group includes family members seeking advice about a service member with a TBI, veterans of previous conflicts, and service members with time-limited needs that do not require continuous tracking. For these individuals, RCCs provide education about TBI, short-term support ("a listening ear"), or contact information for appropriate service providers. These contacts typically complete within one telephone call, but in some cases, RCCs may follow-up with additional information for the caller after doing research to identify the appropriate resources.

Referrals

According to data from CCP, the majority of CCP referrals are received from LRMC (82 percent in 2011; see Figure 4.1). Service members serving in OEF/OIF who experience a traumatic injury that cannot be treated in theater are airlifted to receive initial medical attention and screening at LRMC. While there, all patients undergo extensive neurocognitive testing to evaluate possible TBIs. LRMC forwards to CCP the names, contact information, and locations on redeployment of all service members who screen positive for a mild or moderate TBI and require services. CCP distributes this list to the RCC serving the returning service member's region, and the RCC then contacts the service member directly to describe the program; assess his or her needs; and, when appropriate, invite them to use CCP services. RCCs often described these proactive calls to eligible service members as an important strength of the program, noting that when they call,

> [Service members are often] very grateful, very open to the discussion and receiving help, but based on what they've been through, very overwhelmed, having trouble reaching out themselves.

Similarly,

> So many service members fall through the cracks without someone calling them. You can tell them "call me," but so few of them

Figure 4.1
Referral Sources for 2011 CCP Caseload

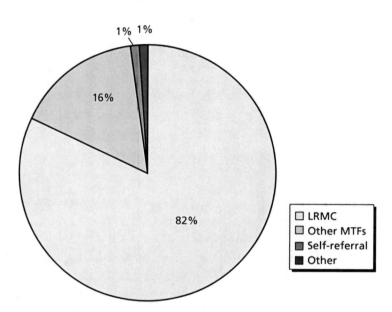

NOTE: Data obtained from DVBIC CCP.

RAND RR126-4.1

do [call] because they're in their day-to-day life. It's hectic. They have memory problems, and they don't think of it.

The LMRC referral process has been an efficient strategy for identifying service members who sustain TBIs in OEF/OIF. However, as these conflicts draw down, this referral source is likely to slow or end. If no other strategy for maintaining caseload is identified, CCP may find itself operating at a significantly smaller scale or may cease to operate altogether. For CCP to remain sustainable, referrals from other sources will need to grow.

After LRMC, the second most common referral source is other MTFs (16 percent in 2011). As part of their job, RCCs reach out to MTFs located in their regions to ensure that providers practicing at these facilities are knowledgeable about CCP and refer eligible service members and veterans who would benefit from the program's services.

The final referral sources, self-referrals and "other," represent only a small fraction of the CCP caseload (2 percent in 2011). To date, service members and veterans or their families have not typically contacted care coordinators directly to seek services. However, program leaders indicate that this is a legitimate route to access. Improving program visibility among service members recovering from a TBI and their families may be one strategy to maintain relevance as fewer new cases are identified directly from conflict zones.

Declining Caseloads

In 2011, this system of recruitment produced a total caseload of 1,129 service members with symptomatic mild or moderate TBI. This caseload represents 4.5 percent of the 24,883 service members diagnosed with a mild TBI in 2011 (DVBIC, 2012b) and likely represents an even smaller percentage of the total number of TBI cases (Hoge et al., 2008; Schell and Marshall, 2008), many of which go undiagnosed. Of course, most cases of mild TBI resolve naturally, without intervention, and would not need or benefit from CCP services. Nevertheless, the discrepancy in the figures suggests CCP may not be reaching the full population of service members who would benefit from program services.

During interviews, RCCs noted that their caseloads have been declining dramatically. Although we lacked access to the data necessary to provide a precise description of the decline, individual RCCs reported declines of as much as 50 percent from their highest caseloads. When queried, they attributed this decline to smaller referral lists from LRMC and to refinement of population eligibility. For example, one RCC noted that,

> It was identified initially that we would follow all TBI diagnoses.
> . . . It wasn't necessarily well defined.

To avoid redundancy with coordination programs serving individuals with severe TBI, the program now focuses on service members with mild or moderate TBI, who would not be eligible for other programs. As the conflicts in Afghanistan and Iraq wind down, fewer service members will be injured and airlifted to LRMC. Given the extent to which CCP relies on LRMC referrals to populate its caseload, one should expect caseloads to drop dramatically in the coming years. However, the program is currently serving only a small proportion of total TBI patients, and therefore, it may be possible to stabilize future caseloads by increasing referrals from other sources. Without swift action, CCP may soon find itself with an insufficient client base. Indeed, at the time of the interviews for this report, some RCCs were already reporting that that they could carry larger caseloads. Engaging underserved eligible service members will be critical in this process.

Avoiding Loss of Services During Transitions and Serving the Underserved

Both administrators and RCCs repeatedly cited their focus on service members who might otherwise "fall through the cracks" as a significant strength of the program. They noted gaps in the clinical care system where service members with a TBI may be lost to follow-up or left without care before they are truly able to manage without support.

Service Members Who Are Transitioning Between Health Care Systems

Many RCCs noted the challenges of transitions:

> Many clients miss the transfer to VA services even though they are given information about the VA while they are in service.

> Where I really see [the program] shine and blossom is the gap when these service members get out of the service.

> When they're in the military, they may or may not have a case manager, but if they do, that stops when they leave the military.

Others identified additional transition points that create risk for losing touch with a service member. For instance, service members experiencing a PCS may require a completely new set of providers. These transition points, when service members are between providers, are moments in which RCC services are perceived as particularly crucial. RCCs' extensive list of nationwide services and their continued relationship with clients before, during, and after transitions, may help smooth these gaps.

Service Members Who Do Not Require More-Advanced Care

Similarly, RCCs see their role as particularly important for service members with a TBI who are not necessarily high-priority patients within other systems. For example, polytrauma centers and the network of federal recovery coordinators ensure that service members with moderate to major injuries receive high-quality care. In many ways, it is fair and equitable that those with the greatest need receive the greatest support. However, this can occasionally mean that service members with mild TBIs are not prioritized for care. DVBIC RCC's identified this underserved group as one they are particularly well equipped to serve:

> The ones that require the most intervention or assistance are the mild ones, because they aren't severe or moderately impaired, so they may not be in the system of care. They may not even have a case manager with the MTF.

During our interviews, we noted both a commitment to serving those with mild TBIs, particularly during transition points, and an indication that the program was nonetheless having trouble finding and accessing this population for services. We outline several of these potentially underserved populations below.

Evacuated Service Members Who Are Not Sent to LMRC

The reliance on the LRMC referral list may inadvertently introduce disparities in access to CCP services. A mild TBI, incurred in a deployed setting, is either treated in the field or, if it requires a higher level of care, prompts transport to the service member's home duty station or a stateside MTF. A mild TBI does *not* trigger a medical evacuation to LRMC (DVBIC, 2012b). Nonetheless, the majority of CCP referrals are for service members evacuated to LRMC who, by definition, must have either a moderate or severe TBI or a mild TBI combined with another primary injury that triggered the evacuation. RCCs are well aware of this limitation and note that

> If they go through Landstuhl [LRMC], the TBI is recorded, tested. But if they're treated in the field by a medic, that's not necessarily going to get recorded and they'll fall through the cracks.

Service members who suffer mild TBIs without an accompanying serious injury are therefore unlikely to come to the attention of the DVBIC CCP, which relies heavily on LRMC referrals. If service members with a mild TBI redeploy to a base with universal TBI screening, such as Fort Carson (Terrio et al., 2009), they may be identified and referred at that point. Service members with mild TBIs who redeploy to bases without screening are likely to miss the opportunity to benefit from CCP services.

Service Members Who Are Not Receiving Treatment at an RCC's DVBIC Site

Officially, RCCs serve any service member with a symptomatic mild or moderate TBI in their four- to ten-state region. In practice, some RCCs report that service members who received treatment at their home institutions make up a disproportionate fraction of the caseload. In many ways, this should be expected. Many RCCs note that the face-to-face contact with providers in their home institution allows them to build strong, professional relationships. Because of such contacts, providers within the RCC's home institution are more likely to refer their TBI cases to the CCP when the service member is ready to discharge from the facility. Providers at another MTF may be unaware of the CCP or have little reason to recall it and are, therefore, less likely to refer their patients to the program. While the process through which such disparities manifest is understandable, the DVBIC CCP has a mandate to serve all service members recovering from a mild or moderate TBI and should consider increasing its efforts to reach service members who happen to receive their medical treatment at a facility other than an RCC's home facility.

Geographically Distant Service Members

RCCs are tasked with outreach to their entire region. However, given constraints in travel funding and difficulty scheduling time away from the office (which necessitates leaving telephones unanswered), many RCCs report that outreach is often concentrated on institutions in their immediate areas. An RCC at an MTF on a large base may communicate with and visit outpatient providers on base and at facilities in the nearest urban center (VA and civilian hospitals and outpatient centers). Therefore, such a coordinator often has a fine-grained, nuanced understanding of the services located within the immediate area around the home office. Similarly, the providers at these facilities may be more likely to have met the RCC and to refer eligible service members when they present, although referrals may still occur at a lower rate than do referrals from providers at the RCC's home facility. One RCC noted that 95 percent of the caseload resided in the immediate area, with only 5 percent residing outside the area, despite the fact that the RCC was officially responsible for service members in a multistate region. The constraints this system introduces mean that service members with a symptomatic TBIs who happen to live in a different state from the RCC, or even in a different region of the state, appear to be less likely to receive CCP services.

Guard and Reserve Forces

RCCs report many of the same challenges reaching Guard and Reserve members as for reaching geographically distant active duty service members. Guard and Reserve members who deploy typically return home to their own communities shortly after returning stateside. The geographic dispersion, possible reliance on civilian health care providers, and limited integration with DoD services may decrease the likelihood that Guard and Reserve members with TBIs are identified for CCP services.

Service Members with TBIs Sustained Outside OEF/OIF

Eligibility criteria for CCP participation include injuries sustained in the Gulf War, OEF/OIF, or Global War on Terror conflicts or during training for these conflicts. Officially, any service member who experiences a non–service related TBI (e.g., a motor vehicle accident, assault, fall) is excluded from the caseload. Service members with TBIs sustained in other conflicts are also excluded. Note, however, that many RCCs will provide referrals and education to callers without adding them to the official caseload.

Innovative Practices and Lessons Learned

The program targets an underserved population (mild TBI). The program's focus on mild TBI captures a population not served by other care coordination programs. Service members with mild TBI might otherwise fall through the cracks of the current military and VA health care system.

Proactive calls engage a population that might not otherwise receive services. RCCs' proactive initial contacts with service members may engage service members who would not otherwise seek assistance but who nonetheless are amenable to help.

Certain program services are available to anyone who calls. RCCs' extensive TBI-related knowledge and skills are not restricted to those service members eligible for services but, rather, are provided freely to any caller who needs help locating support or education about TBI.

CHAPTER FIVE

Outreach and Branding

Outreach to both referral organizations and to individuals who may benefit from the program is considered both an essential feature of the program and a critical factor in its sustainability. Nevertheless, our findings suggest that current outreach and referral strategies may not be reaching certain populations for whom DVBIC CCP services may be beneficial. In fact, outreach was almost uniformly mentioned by RCCs as the one area in which the program could be improved. This includes both direct outreach to potential clients to inform them of the CCP and outreach to DoD, VA, and community-based services to further expand and strengthen the referral network. Below we summarize some of the challenges of program outreach, including lack of name recognition and uniform program presence across DVBIC sites.

The Availability and Accessibility of Funds to Promote Outreach Are Unclear

Several RCCs noted the lack of funds to pay for outreach trips to other states within their regions. They noted that, without such funds, outreach efforts were limited to telephone calls and email, which RCCs viewed as less effective than face-to-face contact. While program leadership reports that each site has a travel budget, it is not clear who manages that budget (i.e., is it the RCC or the DVBIC site administrator?) and whether travel dollars are to be used for outreach efforts or professional development opportunities, such as conference attendance. Some RCCs did note that they use conferences as an opportunity to network and conduct outreach in the city where the conference is located and to network with providers from other sites who are also attending the conference. However, RCCs noted that significant limitations remain. First, only a portion of relevant programs and services may send a representative to the conference. Second, conferences are often held in major cities, limiting opportunities for program exposure in smaller cities and towns, where many service members who may benefit from program services reside. Developing clear protocols for accessing and spending travel budgets may help to clarify these issues and promote outreach within regions.

RCCs Do Not Have Enough Time for Outreach

In discussing outreach efforts with the RCCs, a unifying theme was that they simply did not have adequate time to conduct the amount and quality of outreach that was necessary. As one RCC noted,

> Outreach is not our primary mission, because our primary mission is taking care of the service members on our caseload, but we do need to let people know about us and what we do.

Another noted,

> I would love to have my own outreach coordinator. I have to put my caseload first. If I'm answering phones, how do I go out to the areas in the region?

While focusing on the care coordination of CCP clients is clearly important and should take precedence, findings from Chapter Four suggest that, without a more balanced distribution of time between care coordination and outreach, the program's client base may decline so much that the program is no longer sustainable in its current form. When asked about how outreach may ideally work, RCCs suggested several innovative solutions.

Formalize Collaboration with Regional Education Coordinators

Some RCCs reported partnering with the REC, who is also housed at each site. While outreach for the RCC program is not the REC's job, RECs do travel more frequently and have more contact with both potential clients and service providers, who may provide additional referrals. One RCC expressed a desire to travel with the REC at least once each year around the region to create better networks. Another stated,

> It's really been a challenge with outreach, but I work pretty closely with our educational coordinator. I'll go with him on outreach talks, and he will talk about education, and I'll talk about the RCC program.

This solution may be less than ideal, however, because RECs are currently serving another purpose at DVBIC sites and may not have the time or resources to take on additional CCP outreach duties. Further, in one case, the RCC was also serving as the REC.

Staff at CCP Headquarters Should Lead Outreach Efforts

Some RCCs felt that outreach may be better handled by a program administrator(s) at CCP headquarters. Without an active caseload, this person may have more freedom and flexibility to travel and may be able to leverage DVBIC connections. One or two outreach coordinators stationed at headquarters would also facilitate a unified and consistent program presence across the country.

Hire Lead Outreach RCCs to Manage Outreach Efforts

One novel suggestion was to create and hire multiregion outreach coordinators who would be responsible for outreach to one or more of the current RCC regions. These multiregion outreach coordinators would work closely with the RCCs in these regions and could also travel to visit CCP sites in larger multiregion areas. By making the outreach component of the program slightly more centralized, this model might also help to address some of the issues stemming from the decentralized nature of the program, while retaining the advantages of a decentralized system for care coordination.

It was also suggested that, regardless of which model or combination of models is selected to improve RCC outreach, attention should be paid to the site affiliation of the individual(s) tasked with outreach. It was noted, for example, that not having an institution-connected telephone number may improve a potential client's first impression. Since caller ID often identifies the institution rather than the person calling, some thought it would be beneficial not to have a VA telephone number. "There are some of our veterans who think the VA is good and others think not so good. So a lot of times when they see VA calling them . . . , they won't answer the phone."

There Is a Lack of Specificity, Clarity, and Standardization in How the CCP Is Described

As mentioned earlier, one of CCP's hallmarks is its decentralized design and the authority given to RCCs to assist their region's clients as they see fit. While this approach may be ideal for the unique cases, needs, and situations presenting to the RCCs for services, it may be less than ideal for outreach and program materials. One challenge some of the RCCs highlighted is the lack of specificity and clarity in how program services are described, which makes it difficult for community services, providers, and other case managers to understand the RCC's role or to learn how to use them to case managers' advantage. As one RCC noted, "The program has not clearly advertised how it is unique," and another reported that outreach "is pretty much done on a site-by-site basis." In discussing standardization of materials specifically, one RCC stated,

> We don't have any materials that are standardized in any way to talk about our program, to do the outreach. All of our outreach has been very grass roots, what you can figure out for yourself.

Developing and standardizing program outreach materials at the head-quarters level would not only provide a uniform program presence but also ensure that the messaging was the same across regions.

RCCs felt that two points in particular were not well defined or conveyed: (1) the role of the DVBIC RCC in relation to other case management and care coordination programs and (2) the program's ability to follow individuals with TBI through critical transitions. Many RCCs felt that clarifying these advantages would help convey the ways in which their services complement other services and may benefit staff from these programs by reducing their heavy case loads:

> I'd like to see it streamlined so they know to contact DVBIC as TBI care coordinators. It will benefit them in a way that would take a lot off their caseload. . . . Many case managers don't know that we exist.

> It would be helpful to have a statement of purpose that describes what is expected from the program and from the RCCs. Generally, RCCs aim to be there during service members' transition periods, but the interpretation of what that means is unclear.

Clarifying the program's unique services and providing RCC training in standardized program materials and messaging are also likely to improve outreach, align expectations between the RCCs and clients, and promote collaboration with other professionals who may incorrectly perceive CCP services as duplicative or in competition with the services they provide.

Current Program Name Does Not Capture the Program's Focus or Services

One particular branding challenge is that the program often is referred to loosely as care coordination services, rather than by an official program name. Even within the DVBIC website, the page heading for the program lists "Care Coordination" rather than the "DVBIC Care Coordination Program," which could cause the program to be mistaken for other care coordination services or care coordination more generally. Although program leadership confirmed that "DVBIC Care Coordination Program" is the official name, this name is rarely used in web-based materials or in conversations with administrators or RCCs. Referring to the program by the type of services it offers, rather than by its name, also makes it difficult to discern whether it is a well-defined program that one can access or is a service limited to those already receiving care at DVBIC clinical sites.

Noticeably absent from both the program name (Care Coordination Program) and the title of the care coordinators (RCCs) is any reference to TBI. This is surprising, given that the central feature of this program, and what distinguishes it most from other care coordination programs, is its emphasis on individuals with unresolved TBI. Most felt that not having the phrase "TBI" in their program or job title was causing confusion. Several echoed the sentiment:

> "TBI care coordinator" may be a more appropriate name because of potential confusion with other care coordinators out there.

One RCC noted,

> It can be misleading, because we are TBI care coordinators under the name of regional care coordinators.

Both program leadership and RCCs noted that this issue has been under discussion and that TBI will likely be included in the RCC job titles in the near future.

To add to the confusion, the program does not offer care coordination services in the traditional sense of term. The Agency for Healthcare Research and Quality consensus definition of care coordination notes that it "involves the marshaling of personnel and other resources needed to carry out all required patient care activities, and is often managed by the exchange of information about participants responsible for different aspects of care" (McDonald et al., June 2007). RCCs neither directly coordinate services for a service member (e.g., schedule appointments, coordinate transfer of health records) nor officially facilitate the exchange of information between service providers (e.g., sharing information from specialty providers with the primary care provider in advance of an appointment). Instead, RCCs assess the service member's needs, consult their database of regional service providers, provide the contact information of a provider(s) who is well matched to the service member's assessed needs, and encourage the client to schedule an intake appointment.

For CCP, avoiding "warm handoffs" appeared to be a reasoned, philosophical decision. Both administrators and RCCs note that

> [It is] more empowering. We really want them to be independent, not to make them depend on their injury.

Nonetheless, this philosophy is distinct from typical care coordination programs and could, in principle, lead to multiple difficulties. First, if a referring provider or service member expects traditional care coordination and instead receives a listening ear and a telephone number for a local provider, the mismatch between expectation and reality may lead to dissatisfaction with CCP. Second, confusion between CCP services and traditional care coordination may lead to concerns about duplication of services. Site-based care coordinators may feel that the CCP is infringing on the site's clinical territory, when in fact, the CCP offers a stepped-down, less-intensive support service for patients transitioning to independence. Finally, service members with mild TBI may feel that they do not need intensive "care coordination" and self-select out of the program, when in fact they may have responded favorably to the brief contacts, library-like knowledge of TBI and support services, and emotional support CCP offers. We do not have strong evidence of these concerns in the CCP, but they are issues of which the program should be aware.

CCP's proactive and personalized support, virtual clearinghouse of TBI services, and the extensive clinical knowledge of RCCs is a care model more closely aligned with health coaches than with care coordination. Health coaches use telephone meetings with clients for disease monitoring, address adherence to medical protocols, to provide education, and to teach strategies to improve communication between the client and his or her service providers (Vale et al., 2003; Young et al., 2007). It is possible that such a term as "TBI recovery coach" would mitigate much of the confusion RCCs have observed and perhaps improve the ease and success of outreach efforts.

CCP Has an Inconsistent Web Presence Across DVBIC Sites

One significant challenge is CCP's inconsistent web presence across the websites for each DVBIC clinical site. The web pages for some DVBIC clinical sites highlight care coordination services and describe them in sufficient detail, while the web pages for other DVBIC clinical sites offer limited or no information. Currently, about 1 percent of CCP clients are self-referred. While no data are available to us to clarify how self-, friend-, or family-referred participants learn about the program, we suspect that web searches may be one common route. Providers looking to learn more about the program prior to referring patients may also use such searches. Given the need to expand referral sources in the near future, we sought to evaluate the quality, accessibility, and usability of CCP web content by conducting a content analysis (see Appendix A for detailed methods). While outreach to individuals to promote self-referrals may ultimately include social media campaigns and other novel strategies, it must begin with a strong, traditional web presence in the form of a well-designed website that provides service members and their family members the information they are seeking.

Content Analysis of CCP Web Presence

We conducted the content analysis between April 2 and April 10, 2012. It is possible that involvement with an external evaluation, as well as recent changes in program leadership, may already have prompted program changes in CCP's web presence between the time of our assessment and the publication of this report. Therefore, our findings and recommendations should be considered in light of any recent changes to the websites.

At the time of our analysis, when users first read about the CCP on the general DVBIC website, the sole embedded link took users to an interactive map illustrating the regions each of the 13 regional offices serves. Although this map can be used to access RCC contact information, contact information appeared only if the user made a counterintuitive mouse click on an area within the region of interest, but did not click on the star which was the symbol used to indicate the location of the office in that region. Frequent internet users who navigate intuitively without reading site instructions may have been unlikely to access this critical information. Since the time of this analysis, and prior to the publication of this report, changes have been made to the DVBIC RCC website and contact information for each RCC was easier to find.

From this interactive map, users presumably select the RCC office for the region in which they live. Given the path leading to this map, users may expect the mouse click selecting their region to bring them to a region-specific description of the CCP. This did not occur. Instead, users were linked to the homepage for the entire DVBIC operation in the region, which may or may not mention the CCP specifically.

There was considerable variation in the level of detail featured on the regional DVBIC pages. Some provide detailed descriptions of the CCP program, while others failed to mention the program all together. Even subsequent pages linked to the initial portal did not always provide adequate information about the CCP. One-half of the regional sites did not mention the CCP by name or describe it as a unique program. Users were required to navigate additional links to access information about the CCP in their region, and for some regions, this process did not yield the necessary information.

Eighty-five percent of the regional DVBIC websites included a description, no matter how brief, of the services CCP offers. On one site, the description was a brief phrase—"coordination of other specialty services"—listed along with other services DVBIC offers in that region. However, on six of the 13 sites, the description was sizable (e.g., a two-paragraph description, a bulleted list of services).

All the sites included eligibility criteria for the program. Even sites that did not mention CCP include a description of eligibility for DVBIC services in general, which we counted as being present based on the a priori definitions included in our codebook. Eligibility descriptions were in some cases quite brief (e.g., "service members with TBI and their families") and in other cases exhaustive (e.g., a list of states served by the region and specification of the branches of service served by the program). Note that, in some cases, the eligibility criteria listed on the website may be correct for the DVBIC clinical site but do not accurately reflect eligibility for CCP. For example, both active duty service members and veterans are eligible for CCP, but some sites did not describe veterans as eligible for services.

Only two of the 13 (15 percent) regional CCP websites provided information about how to request services. That is, users who successfully navigated the web content, learned about the program, and believed themselves to be eligible for services, may not have learned that self-referrals are possible or how to initiate one. Only one-third of regional webpages included contact information for the RCC. The absence of readily available contact information erects a barrier that may prevent users from seeking additional information or self-referring.

The web content of all 13 sites includes a prominently displayed logo or seal, which may help to communicate site legitimacy and trustworthiness.

Table 5.1 summarizes the results of the content analysis.

Recommendations

Solutions to outreach problems should be explored. Although insufficient time to conduct outreach was almost universally noted as a challenge, RCCs identified several potential solutions and staffing models that may not only promote outreach but also facilitate a more unified program presence and provide some additional centralization to a decentralized program.

Program name and job titles could be strengthened to reflect program focus more accurately. Though the program name and care coordination titles do not currently reflect the program focus on TBI, both program leadership and RCCs noted that this was an issue undergoing serious consideration and that change would likely occur in the near future to help clarify the program's unique emphasis on TBI.

CCP's web presence could be strengthened to improve outreach and referrals. Despite inconsistent and incomplete information

Table 5.1
Web Content for Each Care Coordination Program Office

	Description of Services	Eligibility Criteria	Requesting Services	RCC Contact Information				Logo Present	CCP Identified
				Name	Address	Telephone	Email		
Camp Lejeune, N.C.	X	X						X	X
Fort Bragg, N.C.	X	X	X		X			X	X
Fort Carson, Colo.	X	X		X				X	X
Fort Hood, Tex.	X	X		X				X	
Naval Medical Center San Diego, Calif.	X	X						X	
San Antonio Military Medical Center, Tex.	X	X						X	X
Walter Reed National Military Medical Center, Md.		X				X		X	
Minneapolis, Minn.	X	X				X		X	
Palo Alto, Calif.	X	X						X	
Richmond, Va.	X	X		X	X	X	X	X	X
Tampa, Fla.	X	X						X	X
Charlottesville, Va.		X						X	
Johnstown, Penn.	X	X	X	X		X	X	X	X
Percent present	84.6	100.0	15.4	30.8	15.4	30.8	15.4	100.0	53.8

about the CCP across DVBIC webpages, the infrastructure for a solid web presence already exists at DVBIC.org, and relatively straightforward changes can be made to the content to ensure it will meet the needs of service members with TBI, their families, and providers.

CHAPTER SIX

Recommendations and Conclusions

The DVBIC CCP addresses a well-documented gap in health care provision for service members with TBI by providing a unique and crucial bridge across systems of care and geographic regions. Our assessment of the program identified a number of innovative practices, summarized at the conclusion of each chapter. Perhaps the most notable strength of the program, as identified by the RCCs, is their focus on identifying and serving individuals who may otherwise fall through the cracks. Unlike other care coordinators or case managers, who are limited in both scope and geographic reach, RCCs are individually and at times collectively able to follow clients as they transition from an inpatient facility to an outpatient facility, as they leave active duty and enter the VA system, as they experience a PCS, and as they return to civilian life after separation from the military. Many service members drop out of services during these critical transition periods, which may be especially challenging for those experiencing TBI because of the cognitive demands and the need to reestablish care in a new setting. Despite many notable program strengths, several key issues were highlighted as potential challenges to future program sustainability and expansion. Below, we summarize these challenges and provide recommendations that may help address these limitations. Of note, several recommendations, particularly those related to outreach, are consistent with prior RAND work on the informational needs of service members affected by TBI and their families (Parker et al., forthcoming), which suggests that some of these recommendations may be applicable beyond CCP.

We recognize that the DVBIC CCP may not be able to implement all these recommendations, but we offer them as ideas for consideration as the CCP is continually improved and refined. It is also possible that awareness of an external evaluation and recent changes in program leadership may have already prompted changes to the program between the time of our assessment and the publication of this report. As a result, some of the recommendations may have been addressed already. Therefore, our recommendations should be considered in light of any recent changes to the program.

Recommendations to Improve the Flow of Information

A number of challenges the RCCs discussed related to the ease with which information flowed across RCCs, health systems, and CCP headquarters. While some RCCs have developed "workaround" solutions to some of these challenges, the program may benefit from efforts to reduce current barriers to information sharing.

Expand opportunities for RCC training across health systems. The structure of the CCP is such that some RCCs are situated in VA sites, others are affiliated with MTFs, and still others are in community settings. Some RCCs come to the program without a solid understanding of the military and VA systems, and while the RCCs are trained more generally on military culture, over time some come to have a disproportionate understanding of one system or another, depending on where they are located. RCCs expressed an interest in gaining a greater understanding of other systems to better appreciate the full system of care and better assist individuals, regardless of whether they are active duty, Reserve or Guard, or veterans. Training specific to these issues and opportunities to visit and shadow RCCs in other systems may prove especially helpful, particularly for newer RCCs or those less familiar with the military.

Facilitate uniform access to relevant medical records and health information. A particularly vexing problem RCCs noted is the lack of uniform access to military health records. While those at MTFs have access to health records via AHLTA, those at VA sites are only able to access the records of patients treated in their VA locations, and those in the community do not have access to any medical records. While this is critically important, we acknowledge that this recommendation is particularly challenging to implement because health records are closely regulated. It may be possible, however, for program and DVBIC leadership to work with DoD and VA leadership to develop a system for modified or limited access to relevant information after permission is received from the client seeking services. RCCs with access to this information emphasized its value in facilitating care coordination services.

Continue to develop centralized data and information-sharing tools. RCCs currently manage or contribute to a number of databases that track caseloads, tasks, and community services and resources. While some of this information is shared with CCP headquarters to facilitate program monitoring, the information is not systematically shared across RCCs. Systematic information sharing may not only ease transfers and warm handoffs of clients who relocate but also promote consultation and joint recommendations from multiple RCCs who may provide different perspectives based on their professional backgrounds or expertise in the DoD or VA systems of care. A more-centralized information-sharing system may also help ensure that tracked health care resources meet some threshold of quality. Although conversations with program leadership and RCCs suggested that efforts were under way to develop such information-sharing tools, particularly for the dissemination of TBI resources, such a system has yet to be implemented.

Recommendations to Improve Standardization of the Care Coordination Program

Continue to address variation across sites related to multiple lines of authority. Due to the unique program structure of the CCP, RCCs face multiple lines of authority, which are often blurred. The relative dominance of these lines of authority also varies significantly across sites. Some RCCs noted additional work requirements for the DVBIC site itself (e.g., additional reporting requirements, committee work), while others had no such additional tasks. Although RCCs did note an improvement in recent months around lines of authority for specific issues or concerns, an overall lack of standardization across sites with respect to these issues remains. Standardizing RCC expectations from the program perspective and clearly conveying these expectations to both the RCC and DVBIC site leadership may help to alleviate confusion and promote RCC satisfaction and consistency in job expectations across sites.

Clarify core features of the program and assess fidelity to them. Perhaps one of the more innovative aspects of this program relates to its model, which has core program features but allows RCCs the flexibility and adaptability to meet the unique needs of service members with TBIs in various settings across the country. A major challenge, however, is the lack of clarity regarding what the core features are and where the leeway in shaping the program on the ground is. For example, administrators and RCCs describe the program as following individuals with TBI for 24 months at predetermined points (three, six, nine, 12, 18 and 24 months). Yet it quickly became clear that RCCs close cases well before the 24-month mark, with the majority closed by the 12-month mark. Although closing cases may be perfectly reasonable (e.g., when clinical issues have resolved), doing so is inconsistent with what was described as a core feature of the program, following up for 24 months. Many RCCs also contacted cases more frequently than the prescribed intervals, particularly in the beginning. Frequency of contact is a good example of an optional feature, where the predetermined points can be viewed as the minimum, or core, number of contacts an individual can expect to receive if they engage with the program. The range of services offered provides another example of lack of clarity about core program features. While helping to coordinate clinical care is clearly a core feature, the program was also described as "helping individuals with whatever they need." For some RCCs, this involved providing assistance looking for educational opportunities, for example, while others focused almost exclusively on clinical care. Clearly defining core program features and regularly assessing RCC fidelity to those features may help the program achieve a more unified presence, provide service members with a more consistent set of services across regions, and align the expectations of individuals engaging with the program at all levels.

Consider the value of the current decentralized, regional system of RCC sites. Conversations with program administrators and RCCs highlighted a mix of advantages and disadvantages associated with the current decentralized system. The five years the program has been in existence likely represent an adequate trial of the current organization. The program may wish to formally revisit the current structure to reaffirm or modify it, particularly in light of recommendations to improve outreach (see next section). Hybrid structures, where multiple RCCs could be colocated, could also be considered to capitalize on the relative strengths of the individual RCCs in terms of background and experience with diverse systems of care (i.e., military, VA, and civilian) and resources.

Recommendations to Improve Outreach

Outreach to both referral organizations and to individuals who may benefit from the program is considered both an essential feature of the program and a critical factor in its sustainability. Given changes to our level of involvement in current conflicts, referrals from LRMC—the primary referral source of the program—are likely to decline over time. However, a number of populations may benefit from the program that are not being reached currently. This section provides a number of recommendations to strengthen program outreach efforts.

Clarify funding available to RCCs to promote outreach. Several RCCs noted that their outreach budgets were insufficient, precluding trips to other states within their regions. Program leadership, however, noted that travel budgets are available at each site. Clarifying the amount of funds available for outreach, the procedures for accessing the funds, and the authorities who must approve the use of the funds will likely improve outreach efforts. If funds are not earmarked for RCC outreach specifically, the program may wish to clarify the amount or relative percentage of the travel budget that should be devoted to program outreach.

Consider alternative staffing models to facilitate outreach. RCCs noted that the primary barrier to outreach is the lack of time they have to conduct it. The RCC's primary responsibilities are care coordination and working with individuals to ensure that their needs are met. RCCs offered a number of recommendations for different staffing models that may promote outreach, including transferring outreach responsibilities to a headquarters administrator, formalizing partnerships with RECs, and hiring a limited number of multiregional outreach coordinators who would work closely with the RCCs in their regions. Hiring more care coordinators with smaller regions is another option, which may facilitate outreach by allowing RCCs to increase the proportion of time spent on outreach while focusing on smaller geographic areas. Regardless of which staffing model or combination of models is ultimately selected, it is clear that outreach requires a substantial investment of personnel time and may require additional staff dedicated to this task.

Develop clear, standardized program materials at the headquarters level that all RCCs can use in outreach efforts. Program materials used for outreach were often described as grassroots efforts, developed by the RCC. This approach results in not one, but potentially 13 different sets of materials, each describing the program services slightly differently, with varying levels of detail and completeness. Program leadership should develop clear, standardized program materials that all RCCs can use in outreach efforts. These materials should

- describe the core features of the program
- clarify what makes the program unique and how it complements more-traditional care coordination or case-management services
- describe eligibility criteria—both for short-term assistance and for longer-term care coordination
- include space for RCCs to insert their names, contact information, and locations
- provide detailed and straightforward instructions for users wishing to self-refer or to refer a family member or client.

Developing these materials at the headquarters level not only provides a unified program appearance but also ensures that the messaging is consistent across sites. Taking the responsibility for developing such materials away from the RCCs permits them to focus on care coordination and outreach.

Consider changing the program name and the job title of RCCs to better align with program services and to reflect a focus on TBI. Noticeably absent from both the program name and RCC title is a reference to TBI. This is surprising, given that the central feature of this program, and what distinguishes it most from other care coordination programs, is its emphasis on individuals with unresolved TBIs. Both program leadership and RCCs noted that they are seriously considering adding TBI to the RCC job title help clarify the emphasis on serving individuals with unresolved TBIs. We also note that the term *care coordination* itself may be misleading or confusing because the program services align more with health coaching than with traditional care coordination. Selecting a program name and job title for the RCCs that accurately reflects the program services and population served will likely help to clarify the unique role that the CCP plays in serving individuals with TBI and may help to engage a wider range of individuals who would benefit from CCP services but do not feel they are in need of care coordination per se.

Create a uniform web presence that is easy to navigate. The CPP currently does not have a unique web presence, a presence distinct from that of DVBIC as a whole. When program-specific content is available, it is intermingled with higher-level information about DVBIC, and links between pages do not always bring users to the expected content. More importantly, many regional sites do not include basic information about program services, eligibility for services, or the process for initiating a self-referral, and most sites do not include full contact information for the RCC. As we recommended for the development of outreach materials, program leadership should take the lead in creating CCP web content that includes all relevant information for the program and can be used uniformly across DVBIC clinical site webpages. In addition, program leadership should do the following:

- Ensure that all DVBIC web pages describe the CCP using the same, consistent language and that this information is provided first, followed by any region-specific information.
- Ensure that contact information for the region's RCC appears in multiple, intuitive locations within the web content. Provide physical addresses, telephone numbers, and email addresses to ensure flexibility for users who may prefer different means of contact.
- Create a web maintenance plan to ensure that content, including regional information, such as RCC names and contact information, is updated in real time to keep information current and accurate.
- Carefully consider literacy and usability issues during content redesign. Be particularly mindful that the target user will be recovering from a mild to moderate TBI and may be experiencing cognitive deficits that interfere with typical tracking of content. Research suggests no more than a fifth-grade reading level for communications to the general public (National Work Group on Literacy and Health, 1998; Weiss and Coyne, 1997).
- Seek internal expertise or an external contractor to optimize the website for search engines. For example, steps can be taken to ensure that the CCP website appears early in a list of search results with general search terms (e.g., "military TBI help").

Leverage additional TBI screening data to identify service members who may benefit from program services and explore opportunities to link surveillance programs with care coordination programs. A unique feature of the CCP is the proactive approach to reaching out to individuals who may benefit from program services. Currently, this approach is feasible because of the program's collaboration with LRMC, which forwards a list of prescreened service members with TBI who may benefit from CCP services. The program may wish to investigate whether there are other sources of screening data that can be used to identify individuals who may benefit from program services. For example, all service members returning from deployment complete the Post-Deployment Health Assessment, which includes a TBI screen. If access to these or similar data were possible, the program might be able to identify and proactively approach a greater number of service members with probable conflict-related TBIs.

Recommendations to Improve the Evidence Base

Given the time and resource constraints of this project, RAND did not conduct an outcomes evaluation and thus makes no claims about the effectiveness of program services or the utility of the program relative to other services. This point is critically important because it is currently not known whether the services RCCs provide have meaningful and positive effects on the lives of service members or veterans and their families. Although RCCs and program staff have received positive feedback about the program from individuals they have served, such sentiments cannot be generalized to the broader population or be used as evidence of program effectiveness.

Evaluate outcomes. Ideally, an outcomes evaluation would compare the short- and long-term outcomes of individuals who received CCP services with the outcomes of individuals with unresolved TBI who did not receive program services. Whether the comparison group is obtained by design, with individuals randomized to receive services or not, or via a convenience sample of individuals who have not engaged with the program, such comparisons are critical for understanding CCP's effectiveness in improving the lives of service members with TBIs.

As part of this evaluation, DVBIC should consider the value of the two years of follow-up. One of the goals of the program is to prevent service members from falling through the cracks during transitions. This goal appears to be contradicted by the practice of closing cases before all scheduled follow-up calls have been completed. By closing cases that appear stable, RCCs may miss the opportunity to support a service member through an upcoming PCS or transition out of the military. Hence, one point of evaluation may be to compare the outcomes of service members working with RCCs who tend to keep cases open for longer periods against those of RCCs who tend to close stable cases.

A final aspect of such an evaluation may include an analysis of program data to examine several points raised in this report, such as geographic clustering of existing clients, disparities in access to program services, and the identification of relatively untapped geographic or demographic markets for program expansion.

Conclusions

TBI is considered one of the signature injuries of the OEF/OIF era, potentially affecting hundreds of thousands of military service members. The nature of the injury, including its cognitive effects and varied recovery trajectories, creates barriers to accessing available health care services. These challenges are especially acute at the boundaries between military, VA, and civilian health care systems, boundaries that cause problems even for those not coping with TBI. DVBIC CCP is an attempt to bridge the gap across systems of care. Analysis of this program identified innovative practices, continuing challenges, and lessons learned. The recommendations provided here suggest strategies for meeting these challenges, while maintaining the benefits possible through this novel approach to care.

Methods for Content Analysis of the CCP Web Presence on DVBIC Websites

As noted in Chapter Five, at the time of our analysis, the CCP had an inconsistent and incomplete web presence across DVBIC sites, which may impede self, family, or provider referrals. To assess the state of the CCP's web presence in 2012, we conducted a website content analysis to document the availability and quality of information about the program. Content analysis "entails a systematic reading of a body of texts, images, and symbolic matter" (Krippendorff, 2004). To identify the content categories of interest, we took the perspective of a service member or family member who was seeking information online about their region's CCP. We expected that these website users would be interested in the following content:

- a description of the program's services
- a description of who is eligible to receive services
- information about how to request services
- contact information for their region's RCC.

In addition, we assessed the following secondary attributes that may promote confidence in the program:

- presence of a logo or seal to establish website credibility
- identification of CCP by name or as a unique program.

The content analysis was conducted between April 2 and April 10, 2012. The data presented here therefore refer to the state of the CCP's web presence in spring 2012. It is possible that involvement with an external evaluation, as well as recent changes in program leadership, may already have prompted program changes in CCP's web presence between the time of our assessment and the publication of this report. Therefore, our findings and recommendations should be considered in light of any recent changes to the websites.

Sampling

DVBIC provides a six-paragraph description of the CCP on its website (DVBIC, 2012a.) Embedded in the description of the program is a link to an interactive map of the United States that illustrates the CCP regions. To the left of the map are links to CCP headquarters, the 15 DVBIC sites,[1] service, and LRMC in Germany. Thirteen of these sites have CCP offices.

To evaluate the available web content for each region's CCP, we followed the link from the national interactive map to each region's CCP webpage. The contents of this webpage *and* the contents of any linked webpages were included in the content analysis. Following the links, we assessed the location and activities web pages, including any additional pages offered for more information, for the following DVBIC locations with a current RCC, as they existed at the time of our review:

- Camp Lejeune, North Carolina
- Fort Bragg, North Carolina
- Fort Carson, Colorado
- Fort Hood, Texas
- Naval Medical Center San Diego, California
- San Antonio Military Medical Center, Texas
- Walter Reed National Military Medical Center, Maryland
- Minneapolis, Minnesota

---

[1] In April 2012, when the content analysis was conducted, Fort Belvoir had not been added as a site.

- Palo Alto, California
- Richmond, Virginia
- Tampa, Florida
- Charlottesville, Virginia
- Johnstown, Pennsylvania.

Codebook

We developed a codebook to operationalize the definition of each code evaluated. Codes were developed to capture website content that a user searching for information about the CCP would find useful (e.g., program eligibility criteria). Table A.1 lists the codes, definitions, and clarifying instructions. Each code was scored dichotomously to indicate that the content was either present or absent in a given region's web presence.

Coding Strategy

Two qualitative coders reviewed the content of the web pages listed above and used the codebook definitions (Table A.1) to identify content that was absent or present in each region's web presence. To assess interrater reliability, we used percentage agreement, rather than Cohen's Kappa statistic, because Kappa is extremely sensitive to small sample sizes and skewed data (e.g., codes where nearly all sites receive the same score), both of which were concerns for these data. Percentage agreement is an alternative indicator of interrater reliability that describes the percentage of coding events in which both coders agreed. Percentage agreement does not account for agreement that would be expected due to chance alone, and therefore, care should be taken in interpreting these values (Cohen, 1960). In this content analysis, percentage agreement ranged from 62 to 100 percent. Disagreement, when it occurred, was reviewed and settled by consensus judgment of the coding and senior research team.

Results

Results of the content analysis are presented in Chapter Five.

Table A.1
Codebook for Content Analysis of Care Coordination Program Web Presence

Code	Definition	Notes
Services offered	Any description, no matter how brief, of CCP services	Example descriptions are "provides education," "monitors progress," "helps coordinate transitions between care levels."
Eligibility criteria	Any description of the population the program serves	Must include at least one additional characteristic beyond having had a TBI (e.g., service member, within specified region).
Requesting services	Website provides directions for how to refer for services	None.
RCC name	Name of the care coordinator associated with the office	If any name is listed, count as present. Not assessed for accuracy.
RCC address	If an address is provided that appears to be associated with the RCC, code as present	In some cases, it may be difficult to determine whether the address corresponds to the DVBIC office or the RCC office specifically. If ambiguous, err on the side of coding present.
RCC telephone	If a telephone number is provided that appears to be associated with the RCC, code as present	In some cases, it may be difficult to determine whether the telephone number corresponds to the DVBIC office or the RCC office specifically. If ambiguous, err on the side of coding present.
RCC email	If an email address is provided that appears to be associated with the RCC, code as present	In some cases, it may be difficult to determine whether the email address corresponds to the DVBIC office or the RCC office specifically. If ambiguous, err on the side of coding present.
Logo present	DVBIC or other logo present (e.g., regional medical center)	None.
CCP identified	Code as present if CCP is identified by a unique name or identified as a unique program	It is not necessary for the name to be "Care Coordination Program."

References

American Congress of Rehabilitation Medicine, "Definition of Mild Traumatic Head Injury," *Journal of Head Trauma Rehabilitation,* Vol. 8, No. 3, 1993, pp. 86–87.

Carroll, Linda J., J. David Cassidy, Lena Holm, Jess Kraus, and Victor G. Coronado, "Methodological Issues and Research Recommendations for Mild Traumatic Brain Injury: The WHO Collaborating Centre Task Force on Mild Traumatic Brain Injury," *Journal of Rehabilitation Medicine,* Vol. 36, 2004, pp. 113–125.

Chu, David, Stephen Speakes, and Emerson Gardner, "DoD News Briefing with Under Secretary of Defense David Chu, Lt. Gen. Stephen Speakes, and Lt. Gen. Emerson Gardner from the Pentagon (News Transcript)," news transcript, Washington, D.C.: Office of the Assistant Secretary of Defense (Public Affairs), January 19, 2007. As of August 7, 2012:
http://www.defense.gov/Transcripts/Transcript.aspx?TranscriptID=3871

Cohen, Jacob, "A Coefficient of Agreement for Nominal Scales," *Educational and Psychological Measurement,* Vol. 20, No. 1, 1960, pp. 37–46.

Defense and Veterans Brain Injury Center, "Care Coordination," web page, 2012a. As of March 1, 2013:
http://www.dvbic.org/care-coordination

———, "DoD Worldwide Numbers for TBI: 2011," 2012b. As of July 16
http://www.dvbic.org/dod-worldwide-numbers-tbi

———, "Medical Evacuation," 2012c. As of July 31:
http://www.dvbic.org/medical-evacuation

Department of Veterans Affairs, *Veterans Health Initiative: Traumatic Brain Injury-Independent Study Course,* Washington, D.C.: Department of Veterans Affairs, Employee Education System, 2010. As of July 26, 2012:
http://www.publichealth.va.gov/docs/vhi/traumatic-brain-injury-vhi.pdf

DVBIC—*See* Defense and Veterans Brain Injury Center.

French, Louis M., Glenn W. Parkinson, and Silvia Massetti, "Care Coordination in Military Traumatic Brain Injury," *Social Work in Health Care,* Vol. 50, No. 7, 2011, pp. 501–514.

Helmick, Katherine, Kevin Guskiewicz, Jeffrey Barth, Robert Cantu, James P. Kelly, Eric McDonald, Stephen Flaherty, Jeff Bazarian, Joseph Bleiberg, Tony Carter, Jimmy Cooper, Angela Drake, Louis French, Gerald Grant, Martin Holland, Richard Hunt, Timothy Hurtado, Donald Jenkins, Thomas Johnson, Jan Kennedy, Robert Labutta, Mary Lopez, Michael McCrea, Harold Montgomery, Ronald Riechers, Elspeth Ritchie, Bruce Ruscio, Theresa Schneider, Karen Schwab, William Tanner, George Zitnay, and Deborah Warden, *Defense and Veterans Brain Injury Center Working Group on Acute Management of Mild Traumatic Brain Injury in Military Operational Settings: Clinical Practice Guideline and Recommendations,* 2006. As of July 26, 2012:
http://www.pdhealth.mil/downloads/clinical_practice_guideline_recommendations.pdf

Hoge, Charles W., Dennis McGurk, Jeffrey L. Thomas, Anthony L. Cox, Charles C. Engel, and Carl A. Castro, "Mild Traumatic Brain Injury in U.S. Soldiers Returning from Iraq," *New England Journal of Medicine,* Vol. 358, No. 5, 2008, pp. 453–463.

Hosek, James, Jennifer Kavanagh, and Laura L. Miller, *How Deployments Affect Service Members,* Santa Monica, Calif.: RAND Corporation, MG-432-RC, 2006. As of August 2, 2012:
http://www.rand.org/pubs/monographs/MG432.html

Independent Review Group on Rehabilitative Care and Administrative Processes at Walter Reed Army Medical Center and National Naval Medical Center, *Rebuilding the Trust,* Arlington, Va., 2007, p. 17. As of August 7, 2012:
http://www.nvti.ucdenver.edu/resources/VETSNET/vol15no2/IRG-Report-Final.pdf

IRG—*See* Independent Review Group on Rehabilitative Care and Administrative Processes at Walter Reed Army Medical Center and National Naval Medical Center.

Jaffee, Michael S., Kathy M. Helmick, Philip D. Girard, Kim S. Meyer, Kathy Dinegar, and Karyn George, "Acute Clinical Care and Care Coordination for Traumatic Brain Injury within Department of Defense," *Journal of Rehabilitation Research & Development,* Vol. 46, No. 6, 2009, pp. 655–665.

Krippendorff, Klaus, *Content Analysis: An Introduction to Its Methodology,* Thousand Oaks, Calif.: Sage, 2004.

McCrea, Michael, Grant L. Iverson, Thomas W. McAllister, Thomas A. Hammeke, Matthew R. Powell, William B. Barr, and James P. Kelly, "An Integrated Review of Recovery After Mild Traumatic Brain Injury (MTBI): Implications for Clinical Management," *Clinical Neuropsychologist,* Vol. 23, No. 8, 2009, pp. 1368–1390.

McDonald, Kathryn M., Vandana Sundaram, Dena M. Bravata, Robyn Lewis, Nancy Lin, Sally A. Kraft, Moira McKinnon, Helen Paguntalan, and Douglas K. Owens, *Closing the Quality Gap: A Critical Analysis of Quality Improvement Strategies*, Vol. 7: *Care Coordination*, Rockville, Md.: Agency for Healthcare Research and Quality, June 2007.

National Work Group on Literacy and Health, "Communicating with Patients Who Have Limited Literacy Skills," *Journal of Family Practice*, Vol. 46, No. 2, 1998, pp. 168–176.

Parker, Andrew M., Lisa S. Meredity, David L. Albright, Rachel M. Burns, and Sarah J. Gaillot, *Informing Current and Former Service Members and Their Families About Traumatic Brain Injury*, Santa Monica, Calif.: RAND Corporation, TR-1123-OSD, forthcoming.

President's Commission on Care for America's Returning Wounded Warriors, *Serve, Support, Simplify*, July 2007. As of August 3, 2012:
http://www.veteransforamerica.org/wp-content/uploads/2008/12/presidents-commission-on-care-for-americas-returning-wounded-warriors-report-july-2007.pdf

Priest, Dana, and Anne Hull, "Soldiers Face Neglect, Frustration at Army's Top Medical Facility," *Washington Post*, February 18, 2007, p. A01.

Riccitiello, Robina, "Iraq: A Marine's Experience of Brain Injury," *Newsweek*, March 16, 2006. As of August 6, 2012:
http://www.thedailybeast.com/newsweek/2006/03/16/casualty-of-war.html

Ruff, Ronald, "Two Decades of Advances in Understanding of Mild Traumatic Brain Injury," *Journal of Head Trauma Rehabilitation*, Vol. 20, No. 1, January–February 2005, pp. 5–18.

Sayer, Nina A., "Response to Commentary: The Challenges of Co-Occurrence of Post-Deployment Health Problems," Washington, D.C.: U.S. Department of Veterans Affairs, Health Services Research and Development Service, 2011. As of March 6, 2013:
http://www.hsrd.research.va.gov/publications/forum/may11/may11-2.cfm

Schell, Terry L., and Grant N. Marshall, "Survey of Individuals Previously Deployed for OEF/OIF," in Terri Tanielian and Lisa H. Jaycox, eds., *Invisible Wounds of War: Psychological and Cognitive Injuries, Their Consequences, and Services to Assist Recovery*, Santa Monica, Calif.: RAND Corporation, MG-720-CCF, 2008, pp. 87–115. As of August 2, 2012:
http://www.rand.org/pubs/monographs/MG720.html

Teasdale, Graham, Gordon Murray, Louise Parker, and Bryan J. Jennett, "Adding up the Glasgow Coma Scale," *Acta Neurochirurgica Supplementum*, Vol. 28, No. 1, 1979, pp. 13–16.

Terrio, Heidi, Lisa A. Brenner, Brian J. Ivins, John M. Cho, Katherine Helmick, Karen Schwab, Katherine Scally, Rick Bretthauer, and Deborah Warden, "Traumatic Brain Injury Screening: Preliminary Findings in a US Army Brigade Combat Team," *Journal of Head Trauma Rehabilitation,* Vol. 24, No. 1, January–February, 2009, pp. 14–23.

VA—*See* Department of Veterans Affairs.

Vale, Margarite J., Michael V. Jelinek, James D. Best, Anthony M. Dart, Leanne E. Grigg, David L. Hare, Betty P. Ho, Robert W. Newman, John J. McNeil, and The COACH Study Group, "Coaching Patients on Achieving Cardiovascular Health (COACH): A Multicenter Randomized Trial in Patients with Coronary Heart Disease," *Archives of Internal Medicine,* Vol. 163, No. 22, 2003, pp. 2775–2783.

Weiss, Barry D., and Cathy Coyne, "Communicating with Patients Who Cannot Read," *New England Journal of Medicine,* 1997, pp. 272–274.

Young, Doris, John Furler, Margarite Vale, Christine Walker, Leonie Segal, Patricia Dunning, James Best, Irene Blackberry, Ralph Audehm, Nabil Sulaiman, James Dunbar, and Patty Chondros, "Patient Engagement and Coaching for Health: The PEACH Study—A Cluster Randomised Controlled Trial Using the Telephone to Coach People with Type 2 Diabetes to Engage with their GPs to Improve Diabetes Care: A Study Protocol," *BMC Family Practice,* Vol. 8, 2007.